MRI of the Musculoskeletal System

Second Edition

The LWW MRI Teaching File Series

SERIES EDITORS

Robert B. Lufkin

William G. Bradley, Jr.

Michael Brant-Zawadzki

MRI of the Brain I

William G. Bradley Jr., Michael Brant-Zawadzki, and Jane Cambray-Forker

MRI of the Brain II

Michael Brant-Zawadzki, Jane Cambray-Forker, and William G. Bradley, Jr.

MRI of the Spine

Jeffrey S. Ross

MRI of the Head and Neck

Robert B. Lufkin, Alexandra Borges, Kim N. Nguyen, and Yoshimi Anzai

MRI of the Musculoskeletal System

Karence K. Chan and Mini Pathria

Pediatric MRI

Rosalind B. Dietrich

The LWW MRI Teaching File Series

MRI of the Musculoskeletal System

Second Edition

Editors

Karence K. Chan, M.D.
Musculoskeletal Radiology
Department of Radiology
Hoag Memorial Hospital
Newport Beach, California

Mini Pathria, M.D.
Professor of Clinical Radiology
University of California at San Diego
School of Medicine
San Diego, California

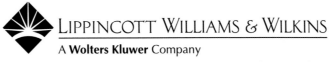

LIPPINCOTT WILLIAMS & WILKINS
A **Wolters Kluwer** Company
Philadelphia · Baltimore · New York · London
Buenos Aires · Hong Kong · Sydney · Tokyo

Acquisitions Editor: Joyce-Rachel John
Developmental Editor: Denise Martin
Production Editor: Kim Yi
Manufacturing Manager: Benjamin Rivera
Cover Designers: David Levy and Jeane Norton
Compositor: Maryland Composition
Printer: Maple Press

©2001 by LIPPINCOTT WILLIAMS & WILKINS
530 Walnut Street
Philadelphia, PA 19106 USA
LWW.com

Printed in the USA

Library of Congress Cataloging-in-Publication Data

MRI of the musculoskeletal system / editors, Karence K. Chan, Mini Pathria.— 2nd ed.
    p. ; cm. — (The LWW MRI teaching file series)
  Includes bibliographical references and index.
  ISBN 0-7817-2571-2
   1. Musculoskeletal system—Magnetic resonance imaging—Case studies. I. Chan, Karence K. II. Pathria, Mini. III. Series.
   [DNLM: 1. Musculoskeletal Diseases—diagnosis. 2. Magnetic Resonance Imaging—methods. WE 141 M93895 2001]
RC925.7 .M752 2001
616.7'07548—dc21

                                                                00-059370

Care has been taken to confirm the accuracy of the information presented and to describe generally accepted practices. However, the authors, editors, and publisher are not responsible for errors or omissions or for any consequences from application of the information in this book and make no warranty, expressed or implied, with respect to the currency, completeness, or accuracy of the contents of the publication. Application of this information in a particular situation remains the professional responsibility of the practitioner.

The authors, editors, and publisher have exerted every effort to ensure that drug selection and dosage set forth in this text are in accordance with current recommendations and practice at the time of publication. However, in view of ongoing research, changes in government regulations, and the constant flow of information relating to drug therapy and drug reactions, the reader is urged to check the package insert for each drug for any change in indications and dosage and for added warnings and precautions. This is particularly important when the recommended agent is a new or infrequently employed drug.

Some drugs and medical devices presented in this publication have Food and Drug Administration (FDA) clearance for limited use in restricted research settings. It is the responsibility of the health care provider to ascertain the FDA status of each drug or device planned for use in their clinical practice.

10 9 8 7 6 5 4 3 2 1

To my parents and my brother Hon, who have sacrificed their lives for my education.

To my husband Barry, whose support helped me achieve my radiology career.

To my teacher, Donald Resnick, who has been a great mentor and friend, providing continuous guidance and encouragement.

Karence K. Chan, M.D.

CONTENTS

PREFACE

The emergence of magnetic resonance imaging (MRI) in the 1980s has changed the way we practice musculoskeletal radiology. Due to its high soft-tissue contrast and multi-planer capability, MRI has played a major role in routine diagnosis of musculoskeletal diseases, including some diseases that were previously undetectable radiographically. Other technical improvements such as newer and faster pulse sequences and the introduction of MR arthrography have markedly increased diagnostic precision. MRI has provided a powerful alternative for a variety of noninvasive procedures including bone scans for evaluating occult fractures and imaging of certain soft-tissue tumors by CT scanning or conventional radiographs. Moreover, MRI has virtually replaced a variety of invasive procedures, thereby changing the course of clinical management and patient care.

This volume illustrates 100 cases of musculoskeletal applications of MRI. The cases are classified into the following categories based on anatomic location: shoulder, elbow, hand/wrist, hip, knee, and foot/ankle. Separate chapters are devoted to arthritis, muscle disorders, and tumor/marrow pathologies. The majority of cases reflect commonly encountered abnormalities; several esoteric examples are also included. A clinical presentation is given for each case, followed by the most relevant radiographic findings, diagnosis, and a brief dicussion of the pathology. Our goal is to provide a basic understanding of the role of MRI in the diagnosis of musculoskeletal disease.

Karence K. Chan, M.D.

ACKNOWLEDGMENT

Our thanks to Robin Francis for her generous and efficient assistance in the preparation of this teaching file.

MRI of the Musculoskeletal System

Second Edition

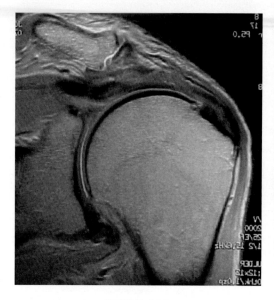

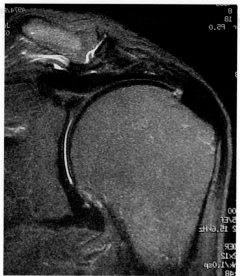

FIGURE 1.1A   **FIGURE 1.1B**

CLINICAL HISTORY

An elderly man fell on an outstretched arm and complained of shoulder pain.

FINDINGS

The oblique coronal proton-density-weighted image shows intermediate signal intensity within the anterior fibers of the distal supraspinatus tendon. The tendon is thinned and irregular approximately 1 cm proximal to its insertion site on the humerus (Fig. 1.1A). On the corresponding T2-weighted image, there is a smaller region of increased signal intensity on the inferior articular edge of the supraspinatus tendon (Fig. 1.1B). There is osteoarthritis of the acromioclavicular joint and a small amount of fluid in the subacromial bursa.

DIAGNOSIS

Partial-thickness tear of the articular surface of the supraspinatus tendon.

DISCUSSION

The rotator cuff is formed by the tendons of four muscles: the supraspinatus muscle superiorly, the infraspinatus muscle superoposteriorly, the teres minor muscle inferoposteriorly, and the subscapularis muscle anteriorly. The rotator cuff reinforces the anterior, superior, and posterior portions of the joint capsule; stabilizes the glenohumeral joint; and functions to abduct and rotate the arm (1,2).

Other than the subscapularis, which inserts on the lesser tuberosity of the humerus, the rotator cuff tendons form a continuous band of attachment along the greater tuberosity of the humerus. The supraspinatus tendon, which inserts on the anterior portion of the greater tuberosity, is most commonly torn. Causes of rotator cuff tear include coracoacromial outlet impingement, trauma, aging, repetitive injury, instability, and systemic disorders that weaken the tendons, such as diabetes, inflammatory arthritis, steroid use, and smoking (3).

Several terms are used to classify tears involving the rotator cuff. A partial tear is present when there is a tear that does not extend through the full thickness of the tendon. Partial tears can involve either the articular or bursal side, though tears of the articular surface are more common (1,3). A full-thickness tear is present when the tear extends all the way through the tendon from its articular surface to its bursal surface. A complete tear is even more extensive and represents a full-thickness tear that extends completely from the anterior to the posterior margins of the tendon.

With MR imaging, coronal and sagittal images are most useful for the diagnosis of a partial tear of the rotator cuff tendons. The presence of definite articular or bursal fluid extending into a portion of the tendon is the most important diagnostic criterion (4). Other findings of partial tear include foci of increased signal within the tendon on T2-weighted sequences. If there are only small foci of high signal, without definite morphologic abnormality of the tendon edge, severe degeneration and tendinitis also need to be considered (1,3). MR arthrography has been suggested as a method to improve the diagnostic sensitivity of MR for partial tears (5).

REFERENCES

1. Resnick D, Kang HS. Shoulder. In: Resnick D, Kang HS, eds. *Internal derangements of joints.* Philadelphia: WB Saunders, 1997:197–209.
2. Otis JC, Jiang CC, Wickiewicz TL, et al. Changes in the moment arms of the rotator cuff and deltoid muscles with abduction and rotation. *J Bone Joint Surg Am* 1994;76:667–676.
3. Tirman PF, Steinbach LS, Belzer JP, et al. A practical approach to imaging of the shoulder with emphasis on MR imaging. *Orthop Clin North Am* 1997;28:483–515.
4. Resnick D. Shoulder imaging. Perspective. *Magn Reson Imaging Clin N Am* 1997;5:661–665.
5. Tirman PF, Bost FW, Steinbach LS, et al. MR arthrographic depiction of tears of the rotator cuff: benefit of abduction and external rotation of the arm. *Radiology* 1994;192:851–856.

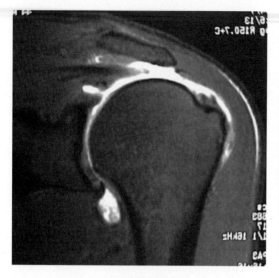

FIGURE 1.2A   **FIGURE 1.2B**

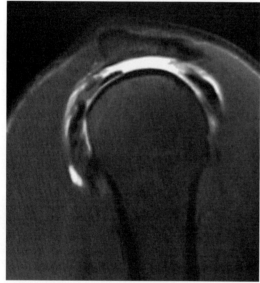

FIGURE 1.2C   **FIGURE 1.2D**

CLINICAL HISTORY

A 44-year-old man complained of shoulder pain.

FINDINGS

Oblique coronal fat-suppressed T1-weighted images (Fig. 1.2A–B) obtained following the intraarticular injection of diluted gadolinium show complete disruption of the supraspinatus tendon (Fig. 1.2A). The fat-suppressed T1-weighted oblique sagittal (Fig. 1.2C) and abduction external rotation (ABER) image (Fig. 1.2D) again show the discontinuity of the supraspinatus tendon. On the sagittal image, note that the anterior portion of the infraspinatus tendon is also torn. The supraspinatus tendon is retracted proximally and a large gap is noted between the proximal and the distal ends of the torn tendon (Fig. 1.2A). Contrast extends from the joint capsule via the tendon disruption into the subacromial and subdeltoid bursa, and subsequently into the acromioclavicular joint (Fig. 1.2B).

DIAGNOSIS

Full-thickness tear of the supraspinatus tendon and the anterior portion of the infraspinatus tendon, with proximal retraction of the supraspinatus tendon.

DISCUSSION

A full-thickness tear of the rotator cuff is defined as a disruption of the tendon that traverses perpendicular to the tendon's long axis, extending from the tendon's articular surface to its bursal surface (1). The most specific signs of a complete tear on MR include complete discontinuity of the tendon with fluid in signal in the gap, retraction of the tendon (2), or absence of the tendon, as can be seen with cases of massive chronic tear (3). Muscular atrophy with fatty replacement is also associated with chronic complete tears. This finding is best seen on T1-weighted images, appearing as linear streaks of high signal within the muscle (2).

Less specific secondary signs of a tear of the rotator cuff are the presence of fluid in the glenohumeral joint, fluid in the subacromial-subdeltoid bursa, irregularity of the tendon, foci of high signal within the tendon, and obliteration of the peribursal fat stripe. However, these secondary signs are less accurate and some of these findings can be seen in asymptomatic individuals. For example, fluid in the subacromial bursa is common even in asymptomatic persons and is frequently present in patients with subacromial bursitis in the absence of a rotator cuff tear. Loss of the peribursal fat is an unreliable finding of a tear and can be seen in many normal individuals, particularly when there is a paucity of body fat.

MR arthrography, which is the term applied to MR imaging performed subsequent to the intraarticular injection of diluted gadolinium, has been found to be more sensitive than conventional MR imaging for detection and characterization of rotator cuff tears, especially for partial articular sided tears of the rotator cuff tendons (4,5). Fat-suppressed T1-weighted images in all three imaging planes are performed immediately following the injection. Utilizing the abduction and external rotation of the arm (ABER position) described by Tirman et al. enhances the detection and characterization of a rotator cuff tear by pooling contrast against the lax articular edge of the tendon (6). In addition to the direct signs of a full-thickness tear that can be identified on conventional MR imaging, the leakage of contrast from the glenohumeral joint into the subacromial-subdeltoid bursa is easily identified and is a very reliable sign of a full-thickness tear (7).

REFERENCES

1. Tirman PF, Steinbach LS, Belzer JP, et al. A practical approach to imaging of the shoulder with emphasis on MR imaging. *Orthop Clin North Am* 1997;28:483–515.
2. Resnick D, Kang HS. Shoulder. In: Resnick D, Kang HS, eds. *Internal derangements of joints.* Philadelphia: WB Saunders, 1997;188–213.
3. Feller JF, Tirman PFJ, Steinbach LS, et al. Magnetic resonance imaging of the shoulder: review. *Semin Roentgenol* 1995;30:224–240.
4. Hodler J, Kursunoglu-Brahme S, Snyder SJ, et al. Rotator cuff disease: assessment with MR arthrography versus standard MR imaging in 36 patients with arthroscopic confirmation. *Radiology* 1992;182:431–436.
5. Palmer WE, Brown JH, Rosenthal DI. Rotator cuff: evaluation with fat-suppressed MR arthrography. *Radiology* 1993;188:683–687.
6. Tirman PF, Bost FW, Steinbach LS, et al. MR arthrographic depiction of tears of the rotator cuff: benefit of abduction and external rotation of the arm. *Radiology* 1994;192:851–856.
7. Tirman PF, Palmer WE, Feller JF. MR arthrography of the shoulder. *Magn Reson Imaging Clin N Am* 1997;5:811–839.

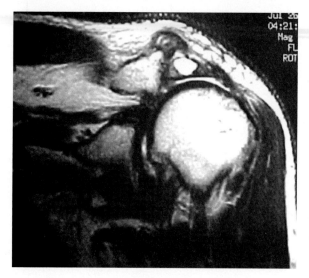

FIGURE 1.3A

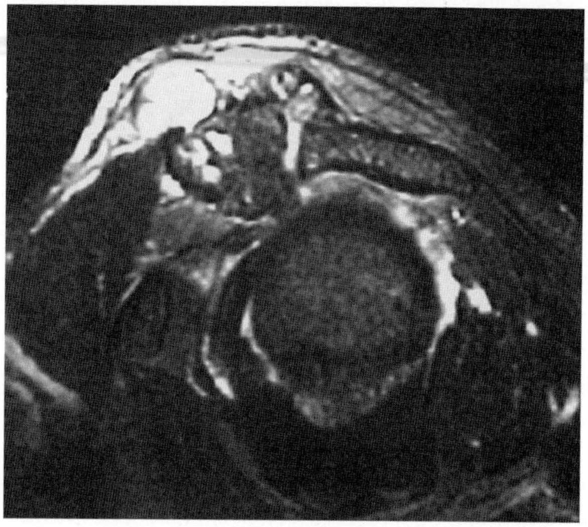

FIGURE 1.3B

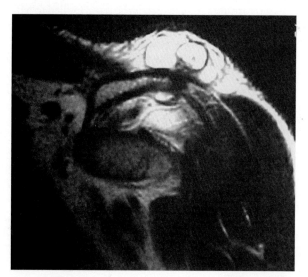

FIGURE 1.3C

CLINICAL HISTORY

A 67-year-old man with pain and a fluctuant palpable mass above his left shoulder.

FINDINGS

The coronal T2-weighted image (Fig. 1.3A) illustrates a complete tear of the supraspinatus tendon, with severe tendon retraction and muscle atrophy. The humeral head is high riding with respect to the glenoid, suggesting a long-standing tear of the rotator cuff. In addition, there is degenerative disease and capsular hypertrophy of the acromioclavicular (AC) joint (Fig. 1.3A). The sagittal fat-suppressed T2-weighted image (Fig. 1.3B) shows severe atrophy of the supraspinatus and infraspinatus muscles and absence of their tendons due to chronic tears. Fluid extends from the glenohumeral joint into the AC articulation (Geyser sign). The sagittal image also shows a multiloculated fluid collection superficial to the diseased AC joint (Fig. 1.3B). The cystic mass, which is well seen on the far anterior coronal T2-weighted image (Fig. 1.3C), produces elevation of the skin adjacent to the AC articulation.

DIAGNOSIS

Complete tears of the supraspinatus and infraspinatus tendons, Geyser sign within an osteoarthritic acromioclavicular (AC) joint, and an associated synovial cyst of the AC joint.

DISCUSSION

Full-thickness tears of the rotator cuff, in the presence of concomitant osteoarthritic changes of the acromioclavicular joint, can result in the formation of an acromioclavicular joint cyst. When the rotator cuff is torn, fluid within the glenohumeral joint fluid can extravasate via the torn rotator cuff into the adjacent subacromial bursa. The bursal fluid can subsequently extend into a degenerated AC articulation if the AC joint capsule is deficient due to severe osteoarthritis (1,2). Continuous communication between the glenohumeral joint and the AC joint causes distension of the AC joint and can ultimately lead to cyst formation (1). The presence of an AC joint cyst usually indicates that there is a massive rotator cuff tear and that the tear is of long standing (1,3). Resection of the AC joint cyst without correcting the underlying rotator cuff pathology typically results in recurrence of the cyst (1,4).

The extension of the fluid from the glenohumeral joint into the acromioclavicular joint and into the AC joint has been termed the *Geyser sign*. The Geyser sign describes the continuous track of contrast fluid extending all the way from the glenohumeral joint into the acromioclavicular joint via the subacromial bursa. The Geyser sign, as well as any associated cyst arising from the AC joint, can be demonstrated by conventional arthrography (3) or by MR imaging (2). On MR, the Geyser sign is best seen on the coronal and sagittal T2-weighted images. If there is an associated cyst, it tends to be multiloculated and can extend for some distance from the AC articulation. The cysts tend to be small because they are easily palpable and present early in the course of cyst formation.

REFERENCES

1. Craig EV. The acromioclavicular joint cyst: an unusual presentation of a rotator cuff tear. *Clin Orthop* 1986;(Jan):189–192.
2. Resnick D, Niwayama G. Internal derangements of joints. In: Resnick D, Niwayama G, eds. *Diagnosis of bone and joint disorders*, 3rd ed. Philadelphia: WB Saunders, 1996:chapter 70.
3. Craig EV. The geyser sign and torn rotator cuff: clinical significance and pathomechanics. *Clin Orthop* 1984;(Dec):213–215.
4. Postacchini F, Perugia D, Gumina S. Acromioclavicular joint cyst associated with rotator cuff tear. A report of three cases. *Clin Orthop* 1993;(Sep):111–113.

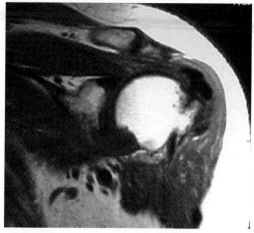

FIGURE 1.4A

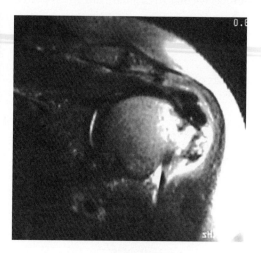

FIGURE 1.4B

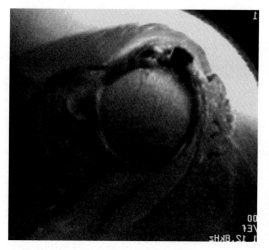

FIGURE 1.4C

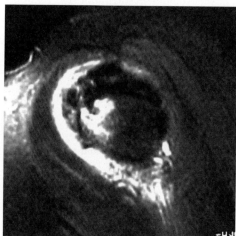

FIGURE 1.4D

CLINICAL HISTORY

A 53-year-old woman had an injury 2 months ago and presented with persistent shoulder pain.

FINDINGS

The oblique coronal T1-weighted (Fig. 1.4A) and fat-suppressed T2-weighted (Fig. 1.4B) images show a bilobed globular mass of low signal intensity both within and superficial to the supraspinatus tendon insertion site (Fig. 1.4A–B). The tendon itself appears intact. The axial fat-suppressed proton-density image again shows a low-signal ovoid density adjacent to the anterior fibers of the supraspinatus tendon (Fig. 1.4C). The lobular low-signal densities are most consistent with intratendinous and peritendinous calcification due to hydroxyapatite deposition. These regions of calcification extend into the subdeltoid bursa and cause adjacent bone edema, soft-tissue inflammation, and bursal fluid, best seen on the sagittal fat-suppressed T2-weighted image (Fig. 1.4D).

DIAGNOSIS

Calcific tendinitis and subacromial-subdeltoid bursitis due to intrabursal rupture of supraspinatus tendon calcification.

DISCUSSION

Calcium hydroxyapatite (HA) crystal deposition occurs in the periarticular soft tissue, particularly within the tendons. The tendons of the rotator cuff represent the most common site of HA crystal deposition in the body. HA deposition can be asymptomatic or result in acute calcific tendinitis or bursitis. Acute calcific periarthritis can be extremely painful and is the most common cause of acute pain in the nontraumatized shoulder (1,2). In the shoulder, the most common location for HA deposition is the supraspinatus tendon (3). The exact cause and pathogenesis of HA crystal deposition in periarticular tissues are unknown. Degenerative disease of the tissues, repetitive tendon injury, and familial predisposition have all been proposed as etiologies for this finding (4).

In its initial silent phase, HA crystals are deposited in the substance of the tendons of the rotator cuff. Subsequently, the deposits may be extruded from the tendon into the floor of the bursa (subbursal rupture stage). The crystals can then extrude further and extend from the tendons into the bursa itself (intrabursal rupture stage). More advanced stages include the adhesive periarthritis phase, in which calcific deposits within the tendon are accompanied by bursitis, and the intraosseous loculation phase, in which the crystal deposits extend into the adjacent bone (4).

Calcific deposits within the tendons of the shoulder are readily diagnosed on conventional radiographs. On MR imaging, calcium HA crystals show low signal intensity on all image sequences. When acute inflammation develops in a bursa, the crystal deposits exist in a semiliquid form and may demonstrate heterogencous hyperintensity with interspersed foci of low signal (5). In purely intratendinous calcification, the low signal due to the HA deposition can be difficult to differentiate from a thickened tendon without calcification, though gradient echo sequences will frequently demonstrate the calcification due to blooming on these sequences (6). Acute inflammatory changes in the bursa and adjacent soft tissues result in periarticular edema and bursal fluid, findings readily seen on MR imaging.

REFERENCES

1. Hayes CW, Conway WF. Calcium hydroxyapatite deposition disease. *Radiographics* 1990;10:1031–1048.
2. Rogers LF, Hendrix RW. The painful shoulder. *Radiol Clin North Am* 1988;26:1359–1371.
3. Beltran J, Noto AM, Herman LJ, et al. Tendons: high-field-strength, surface coil MR imaging. *Radiology* 1987;162:735–740.
4. Resnick D, Niwayama G. Calcium hydroxyapatite crystal deposition disease. In: Resnick D, Niwayama G, eds. *Diagnosis of bone and joint disorders,* 3rd ed. Philadelphia: WB Saunders, 1996:chapter 45.
5. Stoller DW, Wolf EM. The shoulder. In: Stoller DW, eds. *Magnetic resonance imaging in orthopedics and sports medicine,* 2nd ed. Philadelphia: Lippincott-Raven, 1996:chapter 9.
6. Resnick D, Kang HS. Shoulder. In: Resnick D, Kang HS, eds. *Internal derangements of joints.* Philadelphia: WB Saunders, 1997;214–219.

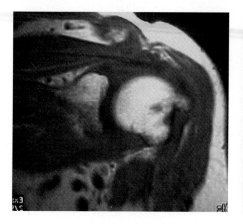

FIGURE 1.5A

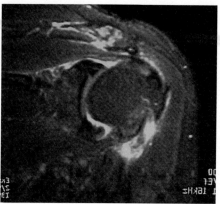

FIGURE 1.5B

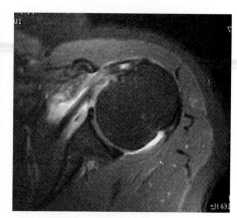

FIGURE 1.5C

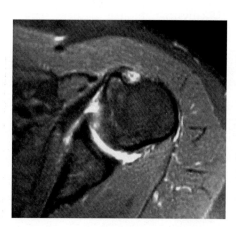

FIGURE 1.5D

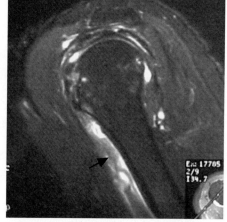

FIGURE 1.5E

CLINICAL HISTORY

A 71-year-old female complained of persistent shoulder pain after a fall.

FINDINGS

The oblique coronal T1-weighted image (Fig. 1.5A) shows intermediate signal intensity in the bicipital groove in the expected location of the low-signal biceps tendon. The oblique coronal fat-suppressed T2-weighted image shows high signal within the biceps tendon proximal to the bicipital groove (Fig. 1.5B). Fat-suppressed proton-density-weighted axial images (Fig. 1.5C–D) reveal a partial tear of the superior fibers of the subscapularis tendon (Fig. 1.5C) and, more distally, absence of normal biceps tendon within the bicipital groove (Fig. 1.5D). The sagittal fat-suppressed T2-weighted image reveals disruption of the biceps tendon with retraction of the tendon distally (Fig. 1.5E, *arrow*). A disproportionate amount of fluid is noted within the bicipital groove as compared with the glenohumeral joint.

DIAGNOSIS

Rupture of the biceps tendon and tear of the superior fibers of the subscapularis tendon.

DISCUSSION

The long head of the biceps brachii tendon arises from the bony supraglenoid tubercle of the scapula and the superior glenoid labrum. The tendon extends anteriorly, laterally, and inferiorly around the humeral head to pass into the bicipital groove, which lies between the greater and lesser tuberosities of the humerus. The normal tendon is best seen on the axial images at the level of the humeral tuberosities as a low-signal oval structure contained within the bicipital groove. Displacement of absence of the tendon can be well visualized on MR imaging at this level. These portions of the tendon are intraarticular, so small amounts of fluid around the tendon are normal in this area, particularly in the presence of a joint effusion.

Further caudally, the biceps tendon emerges from the joint at the lower portion of the groove and is surrounded by a synovial sheath that communicates with the glenohumeral joint (1,2). The major restraint of the tendon within the bicipital groove is the medial coracohumeral ligament. This ligament merges with the subscapularis tendon, which inserts into the lesser tuberosity. Distally, the tendon is restrained by the falciform ligament, the tendinous expansion of the sternocostal insertion of the pectoralis major, and the less important transverse humeral ligament (1).

Disorders of the biceps tendon include tendinitis, tendon subluxation or dislocation, tendon degeneration, and tendon rupture. Tendinitis is typically due to tendon calcification, impingement syndrome, or trauma to the tendon. Patients with acute tendinitis demonstrate synovitis, with synovial thickening and fluid within a distending bicipital tendon sheath. Medial subluxation or dislocation of the biceps tendon is seen in association with tears of the rotator cuff, particularly the subscapularis tendon, or tears of the coracohumeral ligament (2).

Rupture of the biceps tendon may be acute or chronic and is usually seen in association with a coexisting rotator cuff tear (3). The most common site of rupture is at the tendon origin, followed by the site of the tendon's exit from the joint capsule (4). Diagnosis is difficult when the ruptured tendon reattaches within the bicipital groove. MR findings of the rupture of the long head of the biceps tendon include thickening and distortion of the synovial sheath, fluid within the bicipital sheath, absence of the tendon within the bicipital groove, and retraction of the tendon (5). In chronic tears, atrophy and retraction of the tendon can be seen (4).

REFERENCES

1. Ptasznik R, Hennessy O. Abnormalities of the biceps tendon of the shoulder: sonographic findings. *AJR* 1995;164:409–414.
2. Curtis AS, Snyder SJ. Evaluation and treatment of biceps tendon pathology. *Orthop Clin North Am* 1993;24:33–43.
3. Erickson SJ, Fitzgerald SW, Quinn SF, et al. Long bicipital tendon of the shoulder: normal anatomy and pathologic findings on MR imaging. *AJR* 1992;158:1091–1096.
4. Tuckman GA. Abnormalities of the long head of the biceps tendon of the shoulder: MR imaging findings. *AJR* 1994;163:1183–1188.
5. Resnick D, Kang HS. Shoulder. In: Resnick D, Kang HS, eds. *Internal derangements of joints.* Philadelphia: WB Saunders, 1997:299–301.

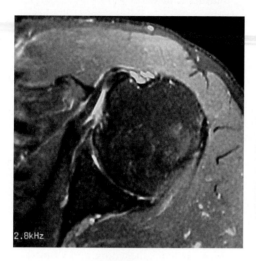 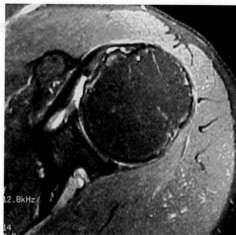

FIGURE 1.6A   **FIGURE 1.6B**

CLINICAL HISTORY

A 51-year-old male with shoulder pain.

FINDINGS

The axial fat-suppressed T2-weighted images (Fig. 1.6A–B) illustrate absence of the normal low-signal tendon of the long head of the biceps brachii in the bicipital groove. The biceps tendon, which is normally located between the greater and lesser tuberosities, has slipped medially to overlie the lesser tuberosity (Fig. 1.6A–B). In addition, the axial images show that the subscapularis tendon is detached from its normal insertion site on the lesser tuberosity.

DIAGNOSIS

Medial dislocation of the long head of the biceps brachii tendon with tear of the subscapularis tendon.

DISCUSSION

Although dislocation of the long head of the biceps brachii tendon can be an isolated finding, almost all cases of dislocation of this structure are due to disruption of its overlying restraining soft tissues, particularly the subscapularis tendon and the medial coracohumeral ligament (1,2). Other predisposing factors include hypoplasia and dysplasia of the bicipital groove, and developmental deficiency of the capsular and ligamentous structures (3). Owing to the orientation of the forces applied on the long head of the tendon, all dislocations result in the tendon displacing medially, to overlie or rest medial to the lesser tuberosity (1,4).

The dislocated biceps tendon can lie superficial or deep to the subscapularis tendon, depending on the integrity of the subscapularis tendon and its attachment to the lesser tuberosity. When the subscapularis tendon is torn, the biceps tendon dislocation is typically deep to the subscapularis tendon. The tendon may dislocate far medially and lie within the anterior aspect of the glenohumeral joint, where it is subject to impingement. In this position, the tendon can simulate a tear of the anterior glenoid labrum. Intraar-ticular dislocation can take place when the subscapularis tendon is intact but has detached from its attachment on the lesser tuberosity. In this situation, the subscapularis tendon insertion at the lesser tuberosity is avulsed but its attachment to the greater tuberosity is still intact (2,4). When the subscapularis is normal, the dislocated biceps tendon lies superficial to the subscapularis tendon and remains extraarticular (5). In this situation, the transverse ligament or coracohumeral ligament is disrupted.

Dislocation of the biceps tendon is commonly associated with a tear of the rotator cuff. The pain produced by the rotator cuff pathology may mask the symptoms from the biceps dislocation, and the diagnosis of biceps dislocation may be missed on clinical examination. Accurate diagnosis by MR imaging is very important given the difference in surgical management (2). The axial image is the best plane for evaluating the relation of the biceps tendon and the bicipital groove and enables delineation of any morphologic changes in the tendon and its supporting structures (6).

REFERENCES

1. Petersson CJ. Spontaneous medial dislocation of the tendon of the long biceps brachii: an anatomic study of prevalence and pathomechanics. *Clin Orthop* 1986;224–227.
2. Chan TW, Dalinka MK, Kneeland JB, et al. Biceps tendon dislocation: evaluation with MR imaging. *Radiology* 1991;179:649–652.
3. Resnick D, Kang HS. Shoulder. In: Resnick D, Kang HS, eds. *Internal derangements of joints.* Philadelphia: WB Saunders, 1997;299–305.
4. Tuckman GA. Abnormalities of the long head of the biceps tendon of the shoulder: MR imaging findings. *AJR* 1994;163:1183–1188.
5. Erickson SJ, Fitzgerald SW, Quinn SF, et al. Long bicipital tendon of the shoulder: normal anatomy and pathologic findings on MR imaging. *AJR* 1992;158:1091–1096.
6. Cervilla V, Schweitzer ME, Ho C, et al. Medial dislocation of the biceps brachii tendon: appearance at MR imaging. *Radiology* 1991;180:523–526.

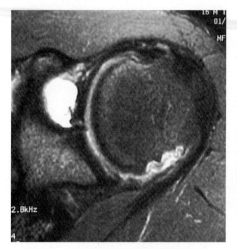

FIGURE 1.7A

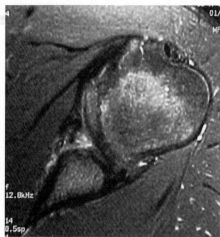

FIGURE 1.7B

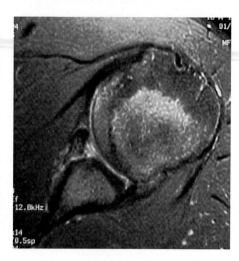

FIGURE 1.7C

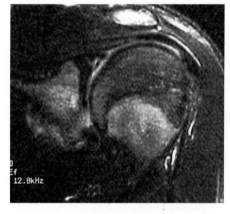

FIGURE 1.7D

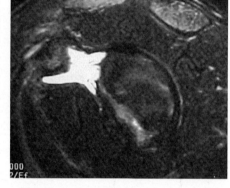

FIGURE 1.7E

CLINICAL HISTORY

A 15-year-old male injured his shoulder while playing sports.

FINDINGS

Irregularity of the posterosuperior aspect of the humeral head is noted on the axial fat-suppressed proton-density-weighted sequence (Fig. 1.7A), consistent with an impaction fracture. In addition, axial, coronal, and sagittal images show that the anterior inferior glenoid bone is fractured (Fig. 1.7B–E). The glenoid fracture fragment is displaced anteromedially. Abnormal linear high signal is seen within the anterior and superior cartilaginous labrum (Fig. 1.7A and D). A large homogeneous fluid collection is presented adjacent to the anterior superior labrum (Fig. 1.7A).

DIAGNOSIS

Sequelae of anterior glenohumeral joint dislocation, with Hill-Sachs fracture of the humerus and Bankart fracture of the glenoid. There is also a glenoid labral tear with associated ganglion cyst formation.

DISCUSSION

Glenohumeral joint instability is a clinical condition defined as symptomatic abnormal movement of the humeral head with respect to the glenoid socket during activity (1). Instability varies from mild subluxation to frank dislocation of the joint. Instability can be classified according to the degree and direction of the instability, the pathogenesis of the disorder, and its chronicity (2). Orthopedists often classify instability into either traumatic unidirectional instability (TUBS) or atraumatic multidirectional bilateral instability (AMBRI) forms (1,3). The TUBS lesion typically has structural abnormalities of the glenoid that require surgery. The AMBRI form is usually managed nonsurgically.

Anteroinferior shoulder dislocation is the most common direction for acute traumatic glenohumeral dislocation. Lesions produced during this dislocation include tears and avulsions of the anteroinferior labrum, tears of the inferior glenohumeral ligament, fractures of the anteroinferior glenoid rim (Bankart lesion), and compression fractures of the posterosuperior humeral head (Hill-Sachs lesion) (4).

On MR, the axial plane is the most useful imaging plane for evaluating the anterior labrum and anteroinferior glenoid. Avulsion of the glenoid rim, labrum, or anteroinferior capsule can be readily identified on the axial images, particularly in the presence of a joint effusion. The avulsed fragment is usually displaced medially and inferiorly due to traction by the inferior glenohumeral ligament (5). Intralabral linear or globular regions of high signal can be seen on the T2-weighted images in the presence of a cartilaginous labral tear. MR arthrography, particularly images obtained with the shoulder in abduction and external rotation, is more accurate for diagnosis of these lesions, particularly in the absence of a joint effusion (6,7).

Hill-Sachs lesions are easily diagnosed on the axial images as well. An area of bony flattening or irregularity is located at the uppermost posterolateral portion of the humeral head, with a maximal inferior extension of 2 cm (8). The Hill-Sachs fracture should not be confused with the normal anatomic groove in the posterolateral portion of the humerus. The most cranial extent of this normal anatomic groove lies between 20 and 32 mm inferior to the top of the humeral head (8).

REFERENCES

1. Tirman PF, Palmer WE, Feller JF. MR arthrography of the shoulder. *Magn Reson Imaging Clin N Am* 1997;5:811–839.
2. Resnick D. Shoulder imaging. Perspective. *Magn Reson Imaging Clin N Am* 1997;5:661–665.
3. Resnick D, Kang HS. Shoulder. In: Resnick D, Kang HS, eds. *Internal derangements of joints.* Philadelphia: WB Saunders, 1997;228–282.
4. Beltran J, Rosenberg ZS, Chandnani VP, et al. Glenohumeral instability: evaluation with MR arthrography. *Radiographics* 1997;17:657–673.
5. Legan JM, Burkhard TK, Goff WBd, et al. Tears of the glenoid labrum: MR imaging of 88 arthroscopically confirmed cases. *Radiology* 1991;179:241–246.
6. Cvitanic O, Tirman PF, Feller JF, et al. Using abduction and external rotation of the shoulder to increase the sensitivity of MR arthrography in revealing tears of the anterior glenoid labrum. *AJR* 1997;169:837–844.
7. Halbrecht JL, Tirman P, Atkin D. Internal impingement of the shoulder: comparison of findings between the throwing and nonthrowing shoulders of college baseball players. *Arthroscopy* 1999;15:253–258.
8. Richards RD, Sartoris DJ, Pathria MN, et al. Hill-Sachs lesion and normal humeral groove: MR imaging features allowing their differentiation. *Radiology* 1994;190:665–668.

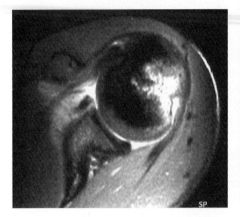

FIGURE 1.8A

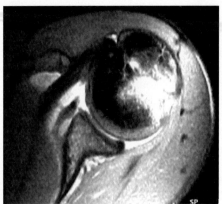

FIGURE 1.8B-1

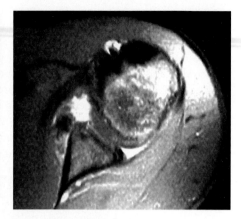

FIGURE 1.8C

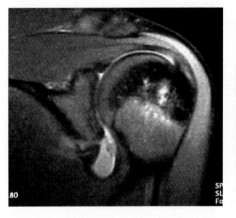

FIGURE 1.8D-1

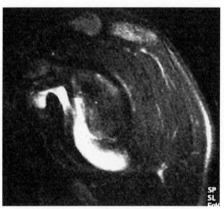

FIGURE 1.8E

CLINICAL HISTORY

A 16-year-old boy with a history of recent shoulder dislocation.

FINDINGS

There is a Hill-Sachs fracture involving the posterolateral humeral head, with surrounding marrow edema (Fig. 1.8A). More caudal axial images (Fig. 1.8B-1–C) demonstrate detachment of the anterior labrum from the glenoid margin with stripping of the periosteum (Fig. 1.8B-2, *arrowhead*). The anterior inferior glenoid rim is fractured and the labrum is internally rotated (Fig. 1.8B-2, *arrow*).

The oblique coronal fat-suppressed proton-density-weighted image again shows the disruption of the inferior glenoid labrum at the site of insertion of the anterior band of the inferior glenohumeral ligament (Fig. 1.8D-2, *arrow*). The sagittal fat-suppressed T2-weighted sequence again shows a defect in the anteroinferior glenoid rim (Fig. 1.8E).

DIAGNOSIS

Anterior labroligamentous periosteal sleeve avulsion (ALPSA) lesion with Hill-Sachs deformity due to anterior dislocation of the glenohumeral joint.

DISCUSSION

In addition to the classic Bankart lesion, a number of variants of anteroinferior labral tears are associated with anterior shoulder instability (1). The ALPSA lesion is one of these variants. In a classic Bankart lesion, there is avulsion of the anterior labroligamentous structures from the anterior glenoid rim, and the anterior capsular periosteum is ruptured, allowing the fracture fragments to separate from the glenoid. In the ALPSA lesion, the anterior capsular periosteum is stripped from the bone but remains intact, holding the avulsed labroligamentous complex down and causing it to rotate inferomedially on the scapular neck (2–4). As a result, the labrum and capsule cannot heal in their normal anatomic position, leading to incompetence of the anterior inferior glenohumeral ligament and recurrent dislocation (2). Differentiation of the ALPSA lesion from a classic Bankart helps preoperative planning of the anterior capsular repair. The surgical approach to these two lesions is different. The ALPSA lesion initially needs to be converted to a Bankart lesion, the fragment reduced, followed by reconstruction of the supporting soft-tissue restraints of the anterior capsule structures (2,4).

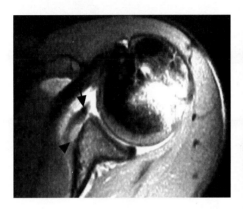

FIGURE 1.8B-2

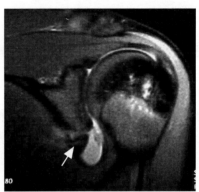

FIGURE 1.8D-2

REFERENCES

1. Beltran J, Rosenberg ZS, Chandnani VP, et al. Glenohumeral instability: evaluation with MR arthrography. *Radiographics* 1997;17:657–673.
2. Neviaser TJ. The anterior labroligamentous periosteal sleeve avulsion lesion: a cause of anterior instability of the shoulder. *Arthroscopy* 1993;9:17–21.
3. Stoller DW. MR arthrography of the glenohumeral joint. *Radiol Clin North Am* 1997;35:97–116.
4. Tirman PF, Palmer WE, Feller JF. MR arthrography of the shoulder. *Magn Reson Imaging Clin N Am* 1997;5:811–839.

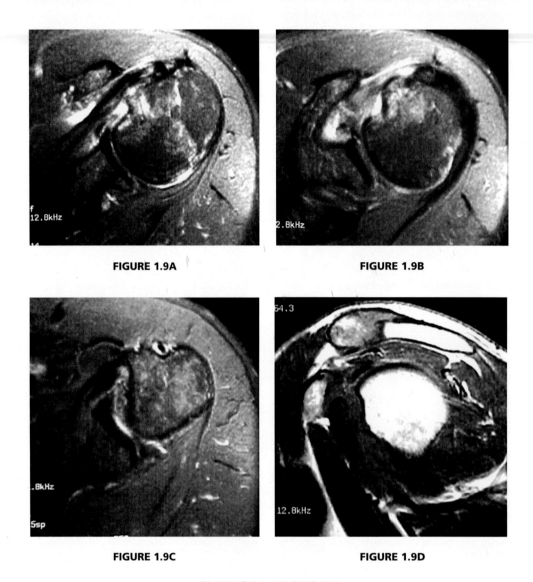

FIGURE 1.9A

FIGURE 1.9B

FIGURE 1.9C

FIGURE 1.9D

CLINICAL HISTORY

A 17-year-old man with a history of a seizure disorder complained of persistent shoulder pain.

FINDINGS

Fat-suppressed T2-weighted axial images of the shoulder show an impaction fracture of the anteromedial humeral head (Fig. 1.9A–B). The more cephalad axial image also shows high signal at the insertion site of the subscapularis tendon (Fig. 1.9A), consistent with a partial tear of the tendon. There is also a fracture of the posteroinferior glenoid rim, separating a fragment of bone and the posteroinferior labrum (Fig. 1.9A–C). The area of humeral flattening is well seen on the T1-weighted sagittal image (Fig. 1.9D).

DIAGNOSIS

Prior posterior dislocation resulting in reverse Hill-Sachs fracture, reverse Bankart lesion, and a tear of the subscapularis tendon.

DISCUSSION

Posterior dislocation of the glenohumeral joint is much less common than anterior dislocation, representing only 2% to 4% of all cases of shoulder dislocation (1). Posterior dislocation most often results from violent muscle contraction due to electric shock or seizure, or due to excessive force applied to the shoulder when the arm is adducted and internally rotated (2,3). The posterior band of the inferior glenohumeral ligament complex is the primary restraint to posterior translation when the shoulder is adducted. During posterior dislocation, the posterior capsular restraints and the posterior labrum may be torn and result in persistent posterior instability (1).

Several bony lesions are associated with posterior glenohumeral instability. When the humeral head dislocates posteriorly, it impacts on the posteroinferior glenoid rim, leading to an impaction fracture of the anterosuperior humeral head, an injury commonly referred to as the trough fracture or a reverse Hill-Sachs lesion. The posterosuperior glenoid rim may be fractured, commonly termed the *reverse Bankart lesion* (2–4). Although these fractures can be identified on conventional radiographs and computed tomography, MR plays an important role in evaluating the capsular, ligamentous, and labral injuries associated with posterior glenohumeral dislocation.

Tears of the posterior capsule appear as a disruption or marked irregularity of the normal continuous hypointense line of the posterior capsule. Posterior capsular disruption at or near the interface with the humerus may also be present. Capsular injury is easiest to identify in the presence of a large joint effusion or following MR arthrography. Fluid or intraarticular contrast extends posteriorly in the planes between the posterior labrum, the capsule, and the infraspinatus muscle (1). Additional associated soft-tissue injuries include edema and hemorrhage within the tendons and muscle fibers of the subscapularis, infraspinatus, and teres minor muscles (1–3).

Injury to the posterosuperior labrum is more difficult to identify than the capsular and tendon injuries. Tears of fraying of the posterior labrum result in absence or contour irregularity of the normal triangular shape of the posterior labrum, or abnormal fluid signal within the labral substance. The labrum may be completely separated from the glenoid. MR arthrography increases the sensitivity of the examination for detection of small and undisplaced posterior labral tears.

REFERENCES

1. Hottya GA, Tirman PF, Bost FW, et al. Tear of the posterior shoulder stabilizers after posterior dislocation MR imaging and MR arthrographic findings with arthroscopic correlation. *AJR* 1998;171:763–768.
2. Beltran J, Rosenberg ZS, Chandnani VP, et al. Glenohumeral instability: evaluation with MR arthrography. *Radiographics* 1997;17:657–673.
3. Tirman PF, Palmer WE, Feller JF. MR arthrography of the shoulder. *Magn Reson Imaging Clin N Am* 1997;5:811–839.
4. Stoller DW. MR arthrography of the glenohumeral joint. *Radiol Clin North Am* 1997;35:97–116.

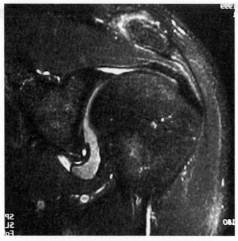

FIGURE 1.10A

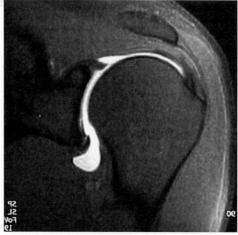

FIGURE 1.10B

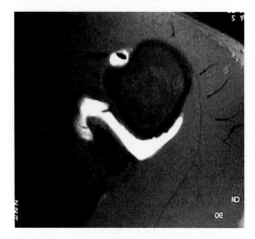

FIGURE 1.10C

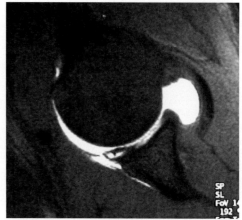

FIGURE 1.10D

CLINICAL HISTORY

This man fell on an outstretched arm.

FINDINGS

On the coronal fat-suppressed T2-weighted image, the anteroinferior labrum shows increased signal (Fig. 1.10A). The coronal fat-suppressed T1-weighted image obtained following MR arthrography with gadolinium shows only subtle linear high signal in the same location (Fig. 1.10B). On the routine axial image, the anterior inferior labrum appears normal (Fig 1.10C). However, when the arm is in the abduction and external rotation (ABER) position, the oblique axial MR arthrogram shows an unequivocal labral tear (Fig. 1.10D). The torn labral-ligamentous complex is displaced away from the bone, and contrast extends into the labrum.

DIAGNOSIS

Anteroinferior labral tear.

DISCUSSION

The glenoid labrum is a ring of fibrous tissue that is present around the entire margin of the glenoid fossa of the scapula. It functions to deepen the glenoid and serves as an attachment site for the glenohumeral ligaments. The peripheral attachment of the labrum joins the capsule and glenohumeral ligaments, forming the capsulolabral complex. The glenoid labrum can be divided into six areas: (a) the superior labrum; (b) the anterosuperior (superior to the midglenoid notch) labrum; (c) the anteroinferior labrum; (d) the inferior labrum; (e) the posteroinferior labrum; and (f) the posterosuperior labrum [1]. The anteroinferior glenoid labral region is most commonly injured, and tears in this region are usually, but not always, associated with shoulder instability. An isolated tear of the labrum can be the cause of shoulder pain without having any clinical sign of shoulder instability [2].

Early diagnosis of an isolated tear of the labrum is important because these tears are symptomatic and have the potential to progress to instability [3]. MR imaging has replaced arthrography and computed tomography for diagnosis of labral lesions because of its higher accuracy and multiplanar imaging capability. The sensitivity of conventional MR imaging varies from 44% to 95%, and the specificity varies from 67% to 86% [4], owing to normal variability in labral size and shape, and difficulty in differentiating a true labral tear from the many normal variations that can be seen within the labrum.

The normal fibrous labrum encircles the peripheral glenoid articular surface and is low signal intensity on all MR sequences. A small amount of hyaline cartilage on the glenoid commonly extends under the base of the fibrous glenoid and should not be mistaken for a labral tear. On the axial images, which show a cross section of the anterior and posterior glenoid, it is usually a triangular or slightly rounded structure [1,5]. The glenoid labrum shows several anatomic variations in its anterosuperior region. In this portion of the glenoid, the labrum may not be attached to the bone or may be separated from the bone by a prominent normal sublabral recess. Although these normal variations can create diagnostic difficulty, they are present in the anterosuperior region and do not involve the anteroinferior glenoid labrum, which is the typical site of labral pathology.

Morphologic MR findings of a labral tear include absence of the labrum, diminution in size, and contour irregularity of its normally smooth margins. A labral tear can also be diagnosed when there are prominent signal alterations within the labrum. Intermediate signal on T1-weighted and proton-density-weighted sequences can be due to myxoid degeneration of the labrum or to magic angle artifact. High signal within the labrum on T2-weighted images indicates the presence of a labral tear. The presence of a perilabral cyst is also a very suggestive finding of a labral tear, even in the absence of any visible abnormality of the labral substance.

With the introduction of MR arthrography, the sensitivity and specificity have improved, owing to distension of the joint with gadolinium-containing agent, which fills the tears and outlines the contours of the deficient labrum. Thus a true tear can be readily distinguished from a pseudotear. In addition, the contrast has higher signal than the underlying hyaline cartilage, which can be separated from a tear [4]. Recently, MR arthrography obtained with the shoulder in the ABER position has been shown to the accuracy of the examination. MR arthrography in the ABER position has a reported sensitivity of 96% and a specificity of 97% for the diagnosis of tears of the labrum [3]. The ABER position exerts a tensile force on the anterior labral-ligamentous complex, particularly on the anterior band of the inferior glenoid labrum, which leads to displacement of the torn fragment from the rest of the labrum. Intraarticular gadolinium can then extend into the displaced tear so that even small tears, as seen in this case, become readily visible [3].

REFERENCES

1. Stoller DW, Wolf EM. The shoulder. In: Stoller DW, ed. *Magnetic resonance imaging in orthopedics and sports medicine,* 2nd ed. Philadelphia: Lippincott-Raven Publishers, 1996:chapter 9.
2. Gross ML, Seeger LL, Smith JB, et al. Magnetic resonance imaging of the glenoid labrum. *Am J Sports Med* 1990;18:229–234.
3. Cvitanic O, Tirman PF, Feller JF, et al. Using abduction and external rotation of the shoulder to increase the sensitivity of MR arthrography in revealing tears of the anterior glenoid labrum. *AJR* 1997;169:837–844.
4. Palmer WE, Brown JH, Rosenthal DI. Labral-ligamentous complex of the shoulder: evaluation with MR arthrography. *Radiology* 1994;190:645–651.
5. Legan JM, Burkhard TK, Goff WBd, et al. Tears of the glenoid labrum: MR imaging of 88 arthroscopically confirmed cases. *Radiology* 1991;179:241–246.

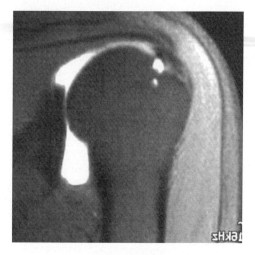

FIGURE 1.11A

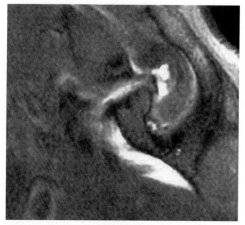

FIGURE 1.11B

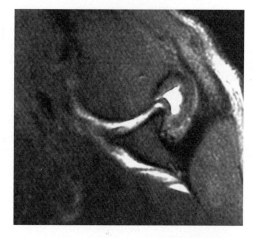

FIGURE 1.11C

FIGURE 1.11D

CLINICAL HISTORY

A baseball pitcher complained of chronic shoulder pain.

FINDINGS

Fat-suppressed T1-weighted images from an MR arthrogram of the shoulder demonstrate cystic changes in the posterosuperior aspect of the humeral head adjacent to the supraspinatus and infraspinatus tendon insertion sites (Fig. 1.11A–B). On the fat-suppressed T1-weighted image in the abduction and external rotation (ABER) position, a linear high signal is present within the posterosuperior labrum with fluid extending into this region (Fig. 1.11C). The articular surface of the supraspinatus tendon is irregular (Fig. 1.11C–D).

DIAGNOSIS

Posterosuperior glenoid impingement syndrome, with tear of the posterosuperior labrum and partial tear of the articular surface of the supraspinatus tendon.

DISCUSSION

Repetitive over-head throwing motion causes abnormal stress on the posterior structures of the shoulder joint. During over-head activities, especially during the late cocking phase of throwing, the humerus is in a position of abduction and external rotation. In this position, the arm angulates posteriorly and the humerus head translates anteriorly within the glenoid. As a result, the undersurface of the rotator cuff contacts and impacts the posterior and superior portions of the labrum and the posterosuperior glenoid (1–3). The repetitive injury to these structures is one of the most common causes of shoulder pain in the throwing athlete (4).

The pathologic manifestations of the posterosuperior glenoid impingement include osteochondral fracture or cystic changes of the posterosuperior aspect of the humeral head, fraying or tearing of the undersurface of the rotator cuff, tearing of the posterior and anterior labrum, tearing of the anterior band of the inferior glenohumeral ligament, and cystic changes within the osseous glenoid (1,4,5).

The osseous changes associated with posterosuperior glenoid impingement can be seen with conventional MR, but the findings of small partial undersurface tears of the supraspinatus tendon and assessment of the posterosuperior labrum can be difficult without adequate distention of the joint with fluid. MR arthrography helps to visualize these lesions, particularly in conjunction with images obtained in the ABER position. The ABER position, obtained with the arm in external rotation and abduction, simulates the position of the shoulder during the cocking phase of throwing. In this posture, the posterohumeral head comes into contact with the posterior labrum and assumes the impingement position. The ABER views have been shown to increase the sensitivity of MR for the detection of undersurface rotator cuff tear and labral tears associated with the posterosuperior glenoid impingement syndrome (6,7).

REFERENCES

1. Roger B, Skaf A, Hooper AW, et al. Imaging findings in the dominant shoulder of throwing athletes: comparison of radiography, arthrography, CT arthrography, and MR arthrography with arthroscopic correlation. *AJR* 1999;172:1371–1380.
2. Davidson PA, Elattrache NS, Jobe CM, et al. Rotator cuff and posterior-superior glenoid labrum injury associated with increased glenohumeral motion: a new site of impingement. *J Shoulder Elbow Surg* 1995;4:384–390.
3. Jobe CM. Posterior superior glenoid impingement: expanded spectrum. *Arthroscopy* 1995;11:530–536.
4. Halbrecht JL, Tirman P, Atkin D. Internal impingement of the shoulder: comparison of findings between the throwing and nonthrowing shoulders of college baseball players. *Arthroscopy* 1999;15:253–258.
5. Tirman PF, Bost FW, Garvin GJ, et al. Posterosuperior glenoid impingement of the shoulder: findings at MR imaging and MR arthrography with arthroscopic correlation. *Radiology* 1994;193:431–436.
6. Tirman PF, Bost FW, Steinbach LS, et al. MR arthrographic depiction of tears of the rotator cuff: benefit of abduction and external rotation of the arm. *Radiology* 1994;192:851–856.
7. Cvitanic O, Tirman PF, Feller JF, et al. Using abduction and external rotation of the shoulder to increase the sensitivity of MR arthrography in revealing tears of the anterior glenoid labrum. *AJR* 1997;169:837–844.

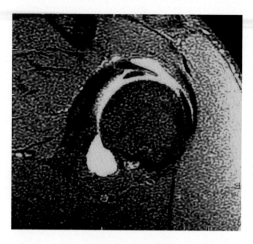

FIGURE 1.12A

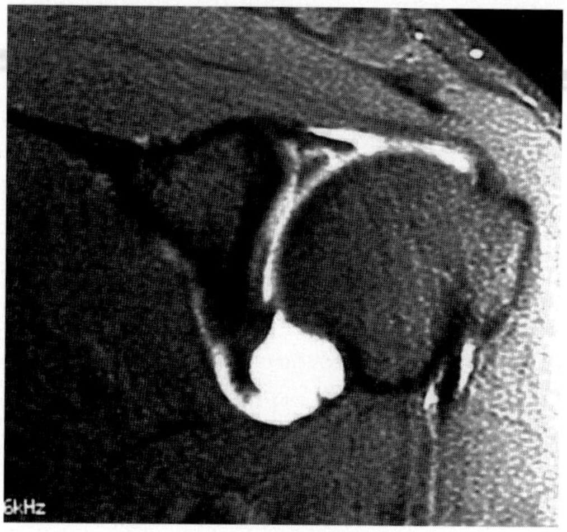

FIGURE 1.12B

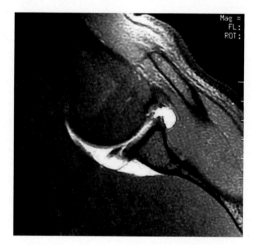

FIGURE 1.12C

CLINICAL HISTORY

This patient has a history of trauma.

FINDINGS

On the oblique coronal fat-suppressed T1-weighted images obtained following MR arthrography, abnormal high signal intensity is noted within the superior labrum immediately below the biceps tendon insertion site (Fig. 1.12A–B). The abnormal signal within the labrum extends anteriorly, as seen on the axial fat-suppressed T1-weighted image (Fig. 1.12C). The biceps tendon and the rotator cuff are normal.

DIAGNOSIS

Superior labral anterior and posterior (SLAP) tear.

DISCUSSION

The SLAP lesion is a tear of the superior labrum at or adjacent to the insertion site of the tendon of the long head of the biceps (1). The injury is usually due to a compressive loading force on the shoulder causing superior subluxation of the humeral head. The superior subluxation causes the humeral head to compress the labrum and biceps tendon, resulting in disruption of the labrum, biceps tendon, and ultimately, the rotator cuff. The SLAP lesion can also be caused by excessive traction applied to the arm and biceps brachii muscle, leading to a tear of the superior portion of the labrum and biceps tendon anchor due to avulsion (1–3).

The most commonly used classification of SLAP lesions divides the tears into four types. More recently, the classification system has been expanded to include as many as nine variants of SLAP lesions (1,4,5). The most commonly used classification describes the SLAP lesion as one of four types, designated as types I to IV (1). The type I lesion is characterized by fraying and degeneration of the superior portion of the labrum. The type II lesion represents separation of the superior portion of the labrum and biceps tendon from the glenoid rim. The type III lesion is characterized by a bucket-handle tear of the superior portion of the labrum with displacement of the labrum away from the bone. The type IV lesion is a bucket-handle tear of the superior labrum with an associated tear extending into the biceps tendon.

The sensitivity of conventional MR imaging for the diagnosis of SLAP lesions, particularly for type I and II variants, has been disappointing. However, the combination of intraarticular injection of the gadolinium-containing agent and MR imaging improves the sensitivity and specificity of the examination for the diagnosis of SLAP lesions (6–8). The MR findings of SLAP lesions include irregular fluid, or contrast agent that extends into the superior portion of the labrum. There may be abnormal widening of the distance between the superior portion of the labrum and the glenoid rim, or a small gap between the superior portion of the labrum that is posterior to the anchor site of the biceps tendon and the glenoid rim (9). Other findings include abnormal high signal intensity that extends into the anterior portion of the labrum and irregular contrast intravasation into the biceps tendon anchor or into the biceps tendon fibers (7).

Submitted by John Healy, UCSD Medical Center, San Diego, CA.

REFERENCES

1. Snyder SJ, Karzel RP, Del Pizzo W, et al. SLAP lesions of the shoulder. *Arthroscopy* 1990;6:274–279.
2. Cartland JP, Crues III JV, Stauffer A, et al. MR imaging in the evaluation of SLAP injuries of the shoulder: findings in 10 patients. *AJR* 1992;159:787–792.
3. Hodler J, Kursunoglu-Brahme S, Flannigan B, et al. Injuries of the superior portion of the glenoid labrum involving the insertion of the biceps tendon: MR imaging findings in nine cases. *AJR* 1992;159:565–568.
4. Maffet MW, Gartsman GM, Moseley B. Superior labrum-biceps tendon complex lesions of the shoulder. *Am J Sports Med* 1995;23:93–98.
5. Resnick D, Kang HS. Shoulder. In: Resnick D, Kang HS, eds. *Internal derangements of joints.* Philadelphia: WB Saunders, 1997;277–278.
6. Flannigan B, Kursunoglu-Brahme S, Snyder S, et al. MR arthrography of the shoulder: comparison with conventional MR imaging. *AJR* 1990;155:829–832.
7. Beltran J, Rosenberg ZS, Chandnani VP, et al. Glenohumeral instability: evaluation with MR arthrography. *Radiographics* 1997;17:657–673.
8. Legan JM, Burkhard TK, Goff WBd, et al. Tears of the glenoid labrum: MR imaging of 88 arthroscopically confirmed cases. *Radiology* 1991;179:241–246.
9. Smith DK, Chopp TM, Aufdemorte TB, et al. Sublabral recess of the superior glenoid labrum: study of cadavers with conventional nonenhanced MR imaging, MR arthrography, anatomic dissection, and limited histologic examination. *Radiology* 1996;201:251–256.

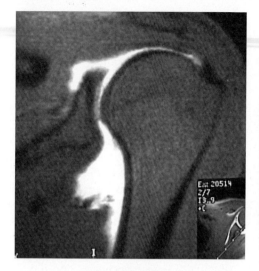

FIGURE 1.13A-1

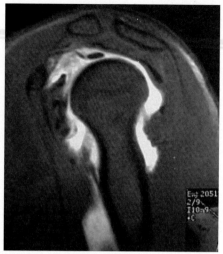

FIGURE 1.13B-1

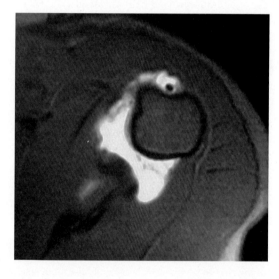

FIGURE 1.13C

CLINICAL HISTORY

An elderly woman complained of chronic shoulder pain. Physical examination elicited findings of anterior glenohumeral instability.

FINDINGS

Coronal (Fig. 1.13A-1), sagittal (Fig. 1.13B-1), and axial (Fig. 1.13C) fat-suppressed T1-weighted images obtained following the intraarticular administration of gadolinium show avulsion of the inferior glenohumeral ligament complex from its humeral attachment site. The contrast has extravasated from the joint via the tear and has extended inferiorly alongside the anteromedial humeral shaft (Fig. 1.13A-2–B-2 *arrowheads*). The glenoid attachments of the inferior glenohumeral ligament are intact (Fig. 1.13B-2, *arrows*).

DIAGNOSIS

Humeral avulsion of the glenohumeral ligament (HAGL) lesion.

DISCUSSION

The HAGL lesion is another cause of traumatic anterior shoulder instability, though it is much less frequent than the Bankart and ALPSA lesions. Unlike Bankart or ALPSA lesions, HAGL lesions tend to occur in an older age group (1,2). The HAGL lesion represents an avulsion of the shoulder joint capsule, including the inferior glenohumeral ligament, from the neck of the humerus. Frequent associated injuries include tears of the subscapularis tendon, dislocation of the biceps tendon, and a Hill-Sachs deformity (3).

Typical MR findings are heterogeneous signal or frank disruption of the anterior capsule at its humeral insertion, and joint fluid extravasation outside the joint between the torn inferior glenohumeral ligament and humeral shaft. MR arthrography is helpful for the diagnosis of the HAGL lesion, especially when there is insufficient joint fluid to demonstrate extravasation from the shoulder joint. Following articular distention with fluid or contrast material, extravasation beyond the joint capsule through the site of avulsion can be readily identified. Accurate diagnosis of the HAGL lesion and appropriate surgical reattachment of the glenohumeral ligament to its humeral insertion will restore anterior stability to the shoulder joint (4).

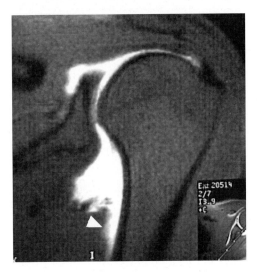

FIGURE 1.13A-2

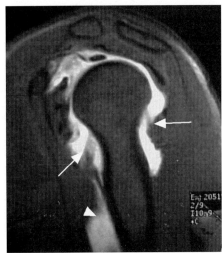

FIGURE 1.13B-2

REFERENCES

1. Feller JF, Tirman PFJ, Steinbach LS, et al. Magnetic resonance imaging of the shoulder: review. *Semin Roentgenol* 1995;30:224–240.
2. Bokor DJ, Conboy VB, Olson C. Anterior instability of the glenohumeral joint with humeral avulsion of the glenohumeral ligament. A review of 41 cases. *J Bone Joint Surg [Br]* 1999;81:93–96.
3. Tirman PF, Steinbach LS, Feller JF, et al. Humeral avulsion of the anterior shoulder stabilizing structures after anterior shoulder dislocation: demonstration by MRI and MR arthrography. *Skeletal Radiol* 1996;25:743–748.
4. Wolf EM, Cheng JC, Dickson K. Humeral avulsion of glenohumeral ligaments as a cause of anterior shoulder instability. *Arthroscopy* 1995;11:600–607.

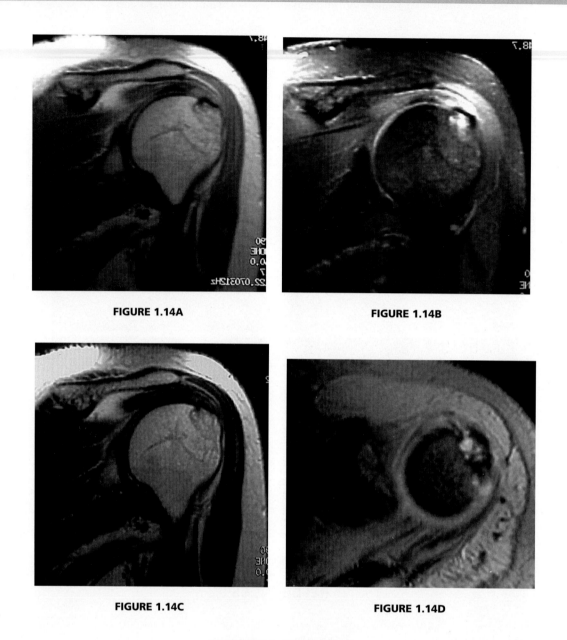

FIGURE 1.14A

FIGURE 1.14B

FIGURE 1.14C

FIGURE 1.14D

CLINICAL HISTORY

A 40-year-old man fell on his left shoulder and complained of severe pain. The radiographs appeared normal.

FINDINGS

Coronal proton-density (Fig. 1.14A) and fat-suppressed proton-density-weighted (Fig. 1.14B) images show an irregular cortex and slight flattening of the greater tuberosity, as well as bone marrow and soft-tissue edema. There is increased signal present within the infraspinatus tendon adjacent to the fracture. On the coronal T2-weighted image (Fig. 1.14C), the inferior surface of the tendon is mildly irregular, but the signal changes within the tendon are much less pronounced. On the axial gradient echo image, cortical disruption and fragmentation of the greater tuberosity are apparent (Fig. 1.14D).

DIAGNOSIS

Undisplaced fracture of the greater tuberosity with intratendinous hemorrhage and partial tear of the infraspinatus tendon.

DISCUSSION

Fractures of the greater tuberosity of the humerus are the result of various mechanisms of injury, most commonly either direct impaction due to a fall or indirect traction forces applied on the greater tuberosity by the rotator cuff. Patients younger than 40 years of age who sustain acute shoulder trauma are more likely to have a fracture of the greater tuberosity than a rotator cuff tear (1). Clinically, these patients present with shoulder pain that is indistinguishable from the symptoms caused by rotator cuff tears (1,2).

When the greater tuberosity is fractured, there may be associated rotator cuff tendinopathy, hemorrhage within the cuff, or a partial tear of the tendon, but a full-thickness tear of the rotator cuff is not commonly associated with a tuberosity fracture. Concomitant injury to the bone and a tear of the rotator cuff appears to be most common in the elderly patient, presumably due to underlying tendinopathy of the rotator cuff tendons.

Since the management strategies for greater tuberosity fracture and acute full-thickness tear of the rotator cuff are different, accurate evaluation of this region is warranted to prevent unnecessary arthroscopy and surgery (2,3). An undisplaced greater tuberosity fracture is treated conservatively, whereas a full-thickness tear of the rotator cuff is treated surgically. A significantly displaced fracture is treated with open reduction and internal fixation to maintain function of the rotator cuff.

Undisplaced greater tuberosity fractures can be very subtle and are easily missed on conventional radiographs, particularly if the patient is unable to rotate the arm externally. These fractures can be confidently diagnosed on MR imaging. A linear low-signal-intensity fracture line can be identified within the tuberosity. Adjacent to the linear fracture line, bone marrow edema of varying degrees is present (3). If the injury is due to impaction, extensive edema may be seen. However, if the fracture is due to avulsion, only a minimal amount of edema may be present (4). The rotator cuff should be carefully evaluated for thickening and increased intratendinous signal, suggesting tendinitis or intratendinous hemorrhage. Following an acute tuberosity fracture, interpretation of high signals within the cuff on T2-weighted images is problematic. Both tendon tears and transient hemorrhage within the cuff produce abnormal high signal on T2-weighted MR imaging. Morphologic alterations, such as irregularity of the tendon margins or thinning of the tendon, are important findings, indicating that a tear is likely. When the tendon only appears thickened, follow-up imaging may be necessary to evaluate the cuff to avoid misdiagnosis of a rotator cuff tear following a fracture.

REFERENCES

1. Zanetti M, Weishaupt D, Jost B, et al. MR imaging for traumatic tears of the rotator cuff: high prevalence of greater tuberosity fractures and subscapularis tendon tears. *AJR* 1999;172:463–467.
2. Mason BJ, Kier R, Bindleglass DF. Occult fractures of the greater tuberosity of the humerus: radiographic and MR imaging findings. *AJR* 1999;172:469–473.
3. Reinus WR, Hatem SF. Fractures of the greater tuberosity presenting as rotator cuff abnormality: magnetic resonance demonstration. *J Trauma* 1998;44:670–675.
4. Palmer WE, Levine SM, Dupuy DE. Knee and shoulder fractures: association of fracture detection and marrow edema on MR images with mechanism of injury. *Radiology* 1997;204:395–401.

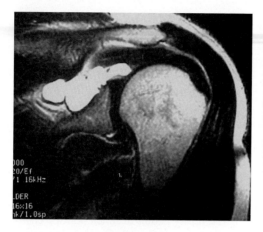

FIGURE 1.15A

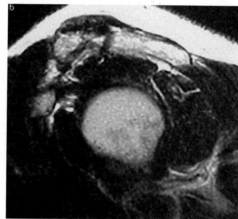

FIGURE 1.15B

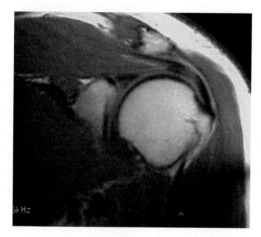

FIGURE 1.15C

FIGURE 1.15D

CLINICAL HISTORY

A 48-year-old man complained of chronic shoulder pain.

FINDINGS

A coronal T2-weighted image of the left shoulder shows a large multilobulated fluid collection in the posterior peri-labral region extending to the suprascapular and the spinoglenoid notches (Fig. 1.15A). On the axial fat-suppressed proton-density image, the fluid collection is again seen posterior to the scapula (Fig. 1.15B). The axial image does not show any definite evidence of a labral tear. On the coronal T1-weighted image, subtle erosion of the bone of the scapular spine can be seen below the cyst (Fig. 1.15C). The sagittal proton-density-weighted image demonstrates mild atrophy of the superior portion of the infraspinatus muscle (Fig. 1.15D).

DIAGNOSIS

Perilabral cyst causing mild atrophy of the infraspinatus muscle.

DISCUSSION

Perilabral cysts of the shoulder are common and are usually associated with an underlying labral tear and glenohumeral instability (1,2). It is hypothesized that fluid from the glenohumeral joint is forced into the surrounding soft tissue through a torn labrum or capsule by a one-way valve mechanism, leading to cyst formation (2,3). Perilabral cysts are strongly associated with an underlying tear of the glenoid labrum, even if such a tear cannot be demonstrated on routine MR imaging. MR arthrography may be necessary to demonstrate a small undisplaced labral tear that is responsible for the formation of the perilabral fluid collection. In most cases, these perilabral cysts communicate with the glenohumeral joint and fill with contrast during MR arthrography. Occasionally, when the tears of the labrum or capsule have completely or partially healed, the communication between the joint and the cyst may be sealed off (1). Large perilabral cysts can cause smooth bone erosion of the adjacent scapula due to pressure on the adjacent bone (2).

On MR imaging, a perilabral cyst can be readily identified due to its high signal on the T2-weighted images. The cyst can be located superior, inferior, anterior, or posterior to the glenoid, depending on the location of the labral tears.

Posterior perilabral cysts are most commonly imaged with MR, possibly because cysts in this location are more likely to become symptomatic due to compression of the suprascapular nerve, which passes through the suprascapular and spinoglenoid notches. The resultant denervation produces pain, weakness, and ultimately, atrophy of the involved muscle.

Compression of the suprascapular nerve produces denervation of the supraspinatus muscle and/or the infraspinatus muscle, depending on the exact location of the cyst. Cysts in the suprascapular fossa compress the nerve proximally and cause denervation of both the supraspinatus and infraspinatus muscles. Cysts located more inferiorly in the spinoglenoid notch compress the nerve distal to the branch innervating the supraspinatus and cause selective denervation of the infraspinatus muscle. Neural compression can result in muscle atrophy. Atrophy of the muscles is identified on the MR imaging by noting decrease in size of the involved muscle and increased fat within the substance of the muscle on T1-weighted images (1,3)

Submitted by Winston S. Whitney, Hoag Memorial Hospital, Newport Beach, CA.

REFERENCES

1. Tirman PF, Steinbach LS, Belzer JP, et al. A practical approach to imaging of the shoulder with emphasis on MR imaging. *Orthop Clin North Am* 1997;28:483–515.
2. Steiner E, Steinbach LS, Schnarkowski P, et al. Ganglia and cysts around joints. *Radiol Clin North Am* 1996;34:395–425.
3. Resnick D, Kang HS. Shoulder. In: Resnick D, Kang HS, eds. *Internal derangements of joints.* Philadelphia: WB Saunders, 1997;306–309.

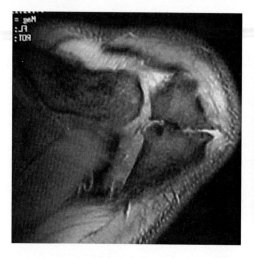

FIGURE 1.16A

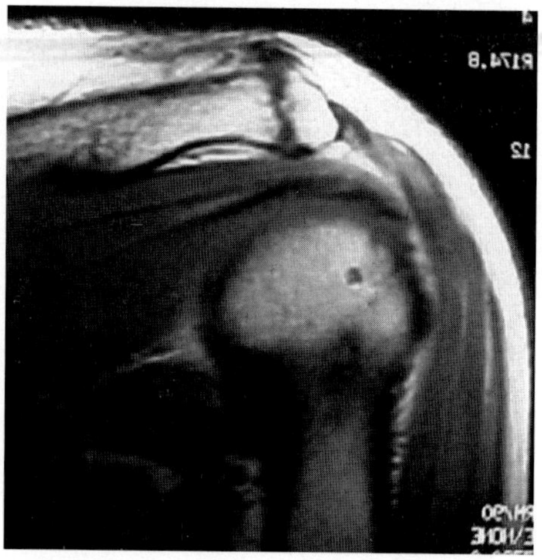

FIGURE 1.16B

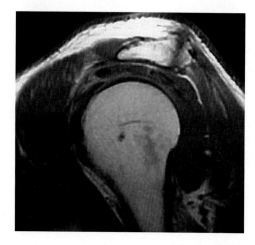

FIGURE 1.16C

CLINICAL HISTORY

A 47-year-old man with shoulder pain.

FINDINGS

The axial gradient echo image shows a coronally oriented cleft with irregular corticated margins in the acromion, just posterior to the acromioclavicular joint (Fig. 1.16A). The sagittally oriented acromioclavicular joint, located antero-medial to the cleft, is normal. The coronal proton-density-weighted (Fig. 1.16B) and the sagittal T1-weighted image (Fig. 1.16C) again demonstrate a vertical low-signal band separating the acromion from the remainder of the scapula. The cleft within the acromion is located posterior to the expected position of the acromioclavicular joint, overlying the infraspinatus tendon.

DIAGNOSIS

Os acromiale.

DISCUSSION

An os acromiale is a developmental abnormality of ossification of the anterior acromion (1). Normally, the anterior ossification center that is present at this location fuses with the remainder of the acromion before 25 years of age. Os acromiale has been classified into seven different types based on the exact location of the unfused ossification centers. The most common types are the mesoacromial and metaacromial variants (1). The case represents the mesoacromial form, which is the most common variant identified with MR imaging.

Os acromiale is typically asymptomatic, but occasionally, the failure of fusion can lead to shoulder pain from abnormal motion at the unfused apophysis (2). Abnormal mobility of the os acromiale can lead to bone marrow edema and the development of a degenerative subacromial enthesophyte at the cleft that impinges upon the underlying tendons, contributing to rotator cuff pathology (1,3). Inferior displacement of the hypermobile ossicle during deltoid contraction further narrows the subacromial space, leading to even more impingement of the rotator cuff. Clinically, the patient may complain of nonspecific shoulder pain and/or pain at marked abduction due to impingement. Point tenderness over the acromion and pain on forward elevation of the shoulder may be detected on physical examination (4).

Preoperative identification of os acromiale prior to acromioplasty for impingement syndrome is important because debridement of the acromion will result in even more instability of a hypermobile ununited acromion. Acromioplasty is contraindicated in the presence of an os acromiale. Instead, surgery is typically performed utilizing open reduction and internal fixation of the os acromion to stabilize the cleft (4,5).

Os acromiale can be identified radiographically, though it is often difficult to visualize without a good-quality axillary view of the shoulder. MR imaging shows the os acromiale well, particularly on the high axial images, and affords concomitant evaluation of the rotator cuff. On T1-weighted MR imaging, a defect of fusion is seen as a low-signal gap orienting in the coronal plane, interrupting the normal high-signal marrow of the distal acromion. On T2-weighted sequences, the signal of the cleft itself varies, depending on the type of tissue present within the fusion defect. The cleft of an os acromiale may contain varying amounts of periosteum, cartilage, synovium, and fibrous tissue (1). When synovium or cartilage is present within the osseous defect, high signal intensity is present on T2-weighted sequences. If the gap is filled predominantly with fibrous tissue, T2-weighted images show low signal. The margins of the gap are low signal because of the presence of corticated bone at the margins of the cleft. The corticated margins are typically irregular or serrated, with overgrowth at the edges of the cleft, similar to the bony changes seen at the margins of spondylolysis in the vertebrae. Bony hypertrophy in the form of a subacromial enthesophyte is often present. Marrow edema may be present when there is hypermobility of the defect. Marrow changes are typically associated with high signal within the cleft as a result of fluid in the interspace.

Although the axial plane is the best plane for evaluation of os acromiale, the oblique sagittal and coronal planes are also helpful, particularly for identifying the associated enthesophyte. On the oblique sagittal plane, a double joint sign can be identified. The os acromiale appears as a pseudoacromioclavicular joint that is located more posteriorly than the normal acromioclavicular articulation. This double joint sign is only present in about 18% of cases of os acromiale due to variability in the exact location of the ossification defect and the exact orientation of the sagittal oblique imaging plane (1).

REFERENCES

1. Uri DS, Kneeland JB, Herzog R. Os acromiale: evaluation of markers for identification on sagittal and coronal oblique MR images. *Skeletal Radiol* 1997;26:31–34.
2. Granieri GF, Bacarini L. A little-known cause of painful shoulder: os acromiale. *Eur Radiol* 1998;8:130–133.
3. Swain RA, Wilson FD, Harsha DM. The os acromiale: another cause of impingement. *Med Sci Sports Exerc* 1996;28:1459–1462.
4. Ryu RK, Fan RS, Dunbar WH 5th. The treatment of symptomatic os acromiale. *Orthopedics* 1999;22:325–328.
5. Warner JJ, Beim GM, Higgins L. The treatment of symptomatic os acromiale. *J Bone Joint Surg [Am]* 1998;80:1320–1326.

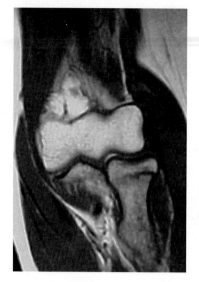

FIGURE 2.17A

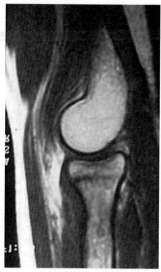

FIGURE 2.17B

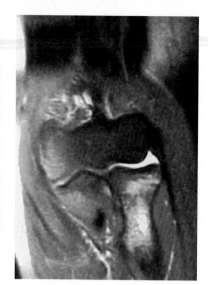

FIGURE 2.17C

CLINICAL HISTORY

A 31-year-old female complained of persistent elbow pain after a fall. Radiographs of the elbow showed only a small effusion within the joint.

FINDINGS

Coronal (Fig. 2.17A) and sagittal (Fig. 2.17B) T1-weighted images demonstrate a transverse low-signal line traversing the radial head-neck junction. Patchy areas of ill-defined low signal intensity are noted in the radial epiphysis, metaphysis, and diaphysis. On the fat-suppressed T2-weighted image (Fig. 2.17C), these areas increase in signal intensity, consistent with edema. A small joint effusion is present.

DIAGNOSIS

Occult fracture of the radial head.

DISCUSSION

Fractures of the radial head are the most common osseous injury in the adult elbow. The most common mechanism for radial head fracture is indirect trauma caused by a fall on the outstretched arm. Less commonly, the fracture is due to a direct blow to the elbow or a severe elbow injury resulting in posterior dislocation of the elbow joint [1,2].

Radial head fractures are classified into three types based on the Mason classification [1]. A type I fracture is a nondisplaced fracture with no angulation or depression. The fracture line may be vertical or horizontal. The type I fracture has an excellent prognosis and is usually managed conservatively. A type II fracture is a marginal fracture where the fracture fragment may be separated, depressed, impacted, or angulated. The type II fracture can be treated conservatively or surgically, depending on the degree of displacement of the fracture fragment. A type III fracture is a comminuted fracture of the radial head. The type III fracture has the poorest prognosis and often results in post-traumatic osteoarthritis of the elbow joint. Because of the extensive comminution of the radial head present in this injury, the type III fracture is usually treated by excision of the radial head. Eppright and Wilkins expanded the Mason classification to include the type IV fracture, in which the injury to the radial head is associated with a dislocation of the elbow articulation. This type of fracture is associated with an even higher complication rate, presumably due to associated soft-tissue injury to the supporting structures of the elbow [1].

Physical examinations are nonspecific in the presence of a fracture of the radial head. Pain, limitation of elbow motion, and swelling are typically present. Accurate diagnosis of a radial head fracture requires an adequate imaging evaluation. On the conventional radiograph, the presence of a fat pad sign due to joint effusion is seen. The radial head and radial neck should be carefully examined for cortical disruption, which can be very subtle in an undisplaced fracture. Computed tomography (CT) is an excellent technique for evaluating fracture morphology and the degree of comminution.

MR imaging is rarely necessary for the diagnosis of radial head fracture. As in other sites in the body, MR can be used to identify an occult fracture in the patient with a posttraumatic elbow effusion and negative or equivocal radiographs. Although detection of radiographically occult fractures is most important in major weight-bearing regions such as the femoral neck, MR can be used in the upper extremity as well. On MR imaging, occult fractures are best seen on a combination of T1-weighted and short tau inversion recovery (STIR) or fat-suppressed T2-weighted images. The T1-weighted sequence shows the orientation of the fracture line and adjacent low signal due to edema. On the STIR and T2-weighted sequences, the surrounding edema becomes bright (3, 4). Although both scintigraphy and MR imaging can detect occult bone injury, the MR examination is more specific because it outlines the anatomic extent of the fracture line.

REFERENCES

1. Weissman BNW, Sledge CB. The elbow. In: Weissman BNW, Sledge CB, eds. *Orthopedic radiology*. Philadelphia: WB Saunders, 1986:190–194.
2. Resnick D, Niwayama G. Physical injury: extraspinal sites. In: Resnick D, Niwayama G, eds. *Diagnosis of bone and joint disorders*, 3rd ed. Philadelphia: WB Saunders, 1996:Chapter 68.
3. Berger PE, Ofstein RA, Jackson DW, et al. MRI demonstration of radiographically occult fractures. *Radiographics* 1989;9:407–436.
4. Stoller DW. The elbow. In: Stoller DW, ed. *Magnetic resonance imaging in orthopedics and sports medicine,* 2nd ed. Philadelphia: Lippincott-Raven, 1996:Chapter 10.

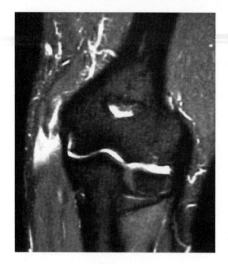

FIGURE 2.18A-1

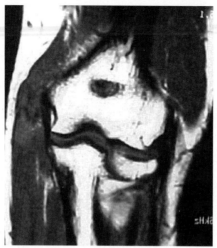

FIGURE 2.18B

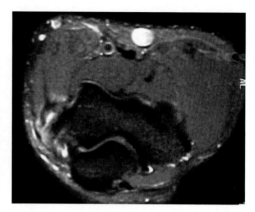

FIGURE 2.18C

CLINICAL HISTORY

A 36-year-old golfer complained of chronic medial elbow pain.

FINDINGS

The coronal fat-suppressed proton-density-weighted image shows increased signal intensity adjacent to the medial epicondyle in the region of the origin of the common flexor tendon (Fig. 2.18A-1–A-2, *arrow*). On the coronal T1-weighted image, the normal low-signal-intensity tendon is intermediate in signal and ill defined, and its attachment to the bone is absent (Fig. 2.18B). The medial collateral ligament, which lies deep to the flexor tendon, remains intact (Fig. 2.18A-2, *arrowhead*). The axial fat-suppressed proton-density-weighted image (Fig. 2.18C) shows high signal intensity at the origin of the common flexor tendon. The tendon is ill defined and irregular.

DIAGNOSIS

Medial epicondylitis.

DISCUSSION

Pain at the origin of the wrist flexor tendon complex at the medial epicondyle of the distal humerus is referred to as medial epicondylitis (1). Medial epicondylitis is also known as golfer's elbow, pitcher's elbow, or medial tennis elbow. It is less common than lateral epicondylitis (2–4). The etiology of medial epicondylitis is thought to be repetitive valgus stress of the elbow, leading to degeneration and tears of the combined origin of the pronator-flexor muscle tendon. Chronic overuse valgus stress not only causes repetitive injury to the common flexor tendon, but also results in injury to the other soft-tissue structures of the medial of the elbow. Medial collateral ligament injury or insufficiency, ulnar nerve tension neuropraxia, as well as intraarticular pathology have all been associated with repetitive valgus injury (3). Initial treatment of medial epicondylitis includes rest, strengthening exercises, and oral nonsteroidal antiinflammatory medications (3). Corticosteroids can be injected at the symptomatic site in recalcitrant patients. If conservative management fails, surgery may be performed to excise the injured areas of the tendon and reconstruct the medial soft tissues.

The diagnosis of medial epicondylitis is based on clinical symptoms and physical examination. However, there may be difficulty in distinguishing medial epicondylitis from medial collateral ligament tear or ulnar neuritis solely on the basis of the clinical evaluation. MR imaging can confirm the diagnosis of medial epicondylitis, evaluate coexisting soft-tissue injury, assess the underlying medial collateral ligament and ulnar nerve, and detect underlying osseous abnormalities (4). The diagnosis of medial epicondylitis is most obvious on T2-weighted sequences because of the presence of high signal within the tendon and adjacent soft tissues. Tendon thickening and increased signal within the tendon are seen on T1-weighted sequences in most patients. In mild cases of medial epicondylitis, the sensitivity of the T1-weighted sequence for the inflammatory changes at the tendon origin is considerably lower than that of the T2-weighted sequences. With more advanced disease, abnormalities in the morphology of the common flexor tendon become apparent. Linear tears can be seen within the tendon in the region of the myotendinous junction. In the presence of a tear, fluid signal intensity can be seen within the tendon on the T2-weighted sequences. Ultimately, the tendon is completely disrupted, leading to the development of a fluid-filled gap within the tendon. The rupture typically takes place in the tendon just distal to the medial epicondyle. Less commonly, the tendon can avulse directly from its osseous site of attachment, leading to edema or osseous avulsion injury of the medial epicondyle.

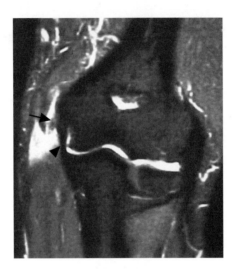

FIGURE 2.18A-2

REFERENCES

1. Martin CE, Schweitzer ME. MR imaging of epicondylitis. *Skeletal Radiol* 1998;27:133–138.
2. Fritz RC, Steinbach LS. Magnetic resonance imaging of the musculoskeletal system: Part 3. The elbow. *Clin Orthop* 1996;Mar(324):321–339.
3. Field LD, Savoie FH. Common elbow injuries in sport. *Sports Med* 1998;26:193–205.
4. Schenk M, Dalinka MK. Imaging of the elbow. An update. *Orthop Clin North Am* 1997;28:517–535.

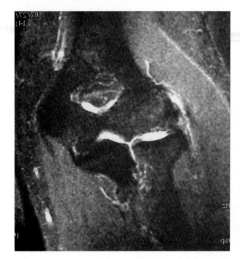

FIGURE 2.19A-1

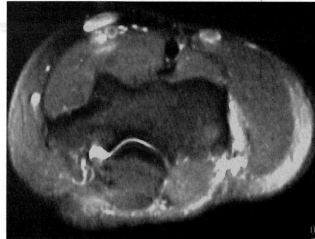

FIGURE 2.19B

CLINICAL HISTORY

A 48-year-old woman had persistent lateral elbow pain.

FINDINGS

The coronal STIR-weighted image (Fig. 2.19A-1) and the axial fat-suppressed proton-density-weighted image (Fig. 2.19B) show increased signal intensity within the common extensor tendon adjacent to its expected insertion site onto the lateral epicondyle. The tendon fibers appear attached to the bone, and there is fluid present adjacent to the lateral epicondyle. There is also high signal present within adjacent muscle. The underlying lateral collateral ligament (Fig. 2.19A-2, *arrow*) appears intact.

DIAGNOSIS

Lateral epicondylitis.

DISCUSSION

Lateral epicondylitis, also known as "tennis elbow," is the most common source of elbow pain in the general population (1,2). The typical age of onset of lateral epicondylitis is the fifth decade of life; males are affected more commonly than females. The diagnosis of lateral epicondylitis is typically made based on the basis of clinical history and physical examination. Clinical symptomatology is characterized by the insidious onset of lateral elbow pain as well as tenderness to palpation in the region of the lateral epicondyle. Most patients can be managed conservatively. Up to 10% of patients

with lateral epicondylitis are resistant to conservative treatment and require surgical intervention (1).

The common extensor muscle and tendon, which arise from the lateral epicondyle of the humerus, is a conjoined tendon arising from several muscles that function to extend the wrist and hand. The extensor carpi radialis brevis tendon, located in the anterior portion of the common extensor tendon, is the most common site of tendon pathology in patients with lateral epicondylitis. Additional tendons that contribute to the common extensor tendon include the extensor digitorum communis, extensor carpi radialis longus, and extensor carpi ulnaris tendons (1). These three tendons are less commonly symptomatic than the extensor carpi radialis brevis. Additional components of the lateral elbow compartment include the supinator muscle and tendon, and the brachioradialis muscle and tendon (3). The lateral collateral ligament of the elbow lies deep to the common extensor tendon. Tear of the lateral collateral ligament complex can occur in association with lateral epicondylitis (3). If the lateral collateral ligament is also torn, the resultant instability of the elbow can be overlooked if the painful overlying tendon lesion precludes adequate clinical assessment.

Lateral epicondylitis is thought to be the result of repetitive injury to the common extensor tendon, either as the result of microtrauma or overuse. Activities that result in repetitive injury to the lateral compartment of the elbow include supinator, brachioradialis, and extensor muscles of the wrist and hand. Histologically, the tendon demonstrates fibrillar degeneration, hyaline and myxoid degeneration, and angiofibroblastic proliferation within the disrupted tendon fibers at its origin. There may be acute or chronic inflammatory changes, but these are variable and not required to make the diagnosis. Since inflammatory changes are inconsistently present, some authors suggest using the term *tendinosis* rather than *tendinitis* to reflect the predominantly degenerative nature of the histologic alterations (1,2).

MR imaging is useful in assessing the degree of tendon damage in those cases of lateral epicondylitis that are resistant to conservative therapy (2,4). Surface coil imaging in all three imaging planes is necessary for adequate assessment of the soft tissues around the elbow articulation. The normal conjoined extensor tendon appears as a low signal on all pulse sequences and has a smooth surface. The attachment of the tendon onto the lateral epicondyle is best assessed on the coronal image, supplemented by the axial plane. The appearance of lateral epicondylitis depends on the degree of tendon abnormality, which progresses from degeneration to the presence of partial or complete tears of the tendon. The T1-weighted sequence demonstrates increased signal intensity within the tendon and does not reliably distinguish degeneration from a frank tear within the substance of the tendon. On T2-weighted or STIR sequence, degeneration remains amorphous low signal, whereas a partial or complete tear shows a focal area of disruption replaced by fluid signal; degenerated tendon shows amorphous signal. Tendon thickening is classically seen in the degenerated tendon, whereas thinning is due to atresia of the tendon and is suggestive of an underlying tear. Edema in the adjacent muscle and soft tissues may be present, particularly in patients with advanced disease.

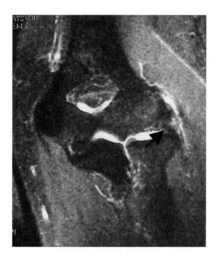

FIGURE 2.19A-2

REFERENCES

1. Field LD, Savoie FH. Common elbow injuries in sport. *Sports Med* 1998;26:193–205.
2. Schenk M, Dalinka MK. Imaging of the elbow. An update. *Orthop Clin North Am* 1997;28:517–535.
3. Fritz RC. MR imaging of sports injuries of the elbow. *Magn Reson Imaging Clin N Am* 1999;7:51–72, viii.
4. Martin CE, Schweitzer ME. MR imaging of epicondylitis. *Skeletal Radiol* 1998;27:133–138.

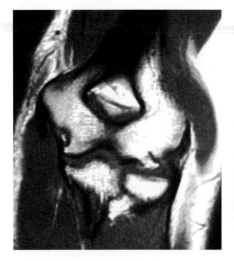

FIGURE 2.20A

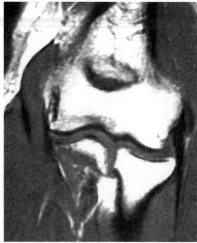

FIGURE 2.20B

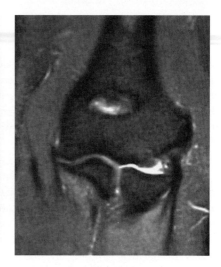

FIGURE 2.20C-1

CLINICAL HISTORY

This young man had lateral elbow pain and a sensation of snapping of the elbow.

FINDINGS

The coronal T1-weighted images (Fig. 2.20A–B) show intermediate signal intensity at the origin of the radial collateral ligament portion (Fig. 2.20A) of the lateral collateral ligament complex. The normal low-signal band of the radial collateral ligament is irregular and is detached from the lateral femoral epicondyle. The overlying common extensor tendon is intact (Fig. 2.20B). On the coronal T2-weighted image (Fig. 2.20C-1), high-signal fluid is seen interposed between the irregular fibers of the radial collateral ligament (Fig. 2.20C-2, *arrow*).

DIAGNOSIS

Tear of the proximal radial collateral ligament.

DISCUSSION

The lateral collateral ligament consists of the radial collateral ligament, the lateral ulnar collateral ligament, the accessory lateral collateral ligament, and the annular ligament. Unlike the medial collateral ligament, which has consistent anatomy, the components of the lateral ligament complex are more variable and less discrete. The radial collateral ligament arises from the anterior lateral epicondyle and broadens as it extends distally to insert onto the annular ligament. The outermost fibers of the radial collateral ligament blend with the overlying common extensor tendon. Posterior to the radial collateral ligament, the lateral ulnar collateral ligament arises from the lateral epicondyle and extends along the posterior aspect of the radius to insert on the supinator crest of the ulna. Both the radial collateral ligament and the lateral lunar collateral ligament stabilize the lateral elbow joint and constraint varus stress. The annular ligament component of the lateral collateral ligament encircles the radial neck and attaches to the anterior and posterior margins of the radial notch of the ulna. The annular ligament is the primary restraint against inferior dislocation of the radial head.

The accessory lateral collateral ligament extends from the annular ligament to the ulna. This ligament is variable and is not always present (1–3).

Injuries of the lateral collateral ligament are less common than those involving the medial side. Patients experience lateral elbow pain with locking and snapping sensations within the joint. Tears of the lateral ligaments are most commonly seen in patients who have sustained elbow dislocation or subluxation, or who injure the ligament due to a hyperextension and varus injury, such as a fall on an outstretched hand. Recently, posterolateral rotatory instability has been emphasized as a common cause of lateral ligamentous insufficiency. Ligament insufficiency has also been reported following a radial head excision or extensor tendon release for lateral epicondylitis (2–5). Repetitive microtrauma from overuse is more commonly associated with lateral epicondylitis than with frank tears leading to insufficiency.

On MR imaging, the coronal plane is best for evaluating the radial collateral ligament and the lateral ulnar collateral ligament, whereas the axial plane is best for visualization of the annular ligament. A sprain of the lateral collateral ligament complex most commonly involves the radial collateral ligament. Ligament sprain manifests on MR as a thickened or thin ligament with high signal in and around its fibers. Once the ligament is torn, irregularity or disruption of the ligament fibers is seen, with increased signal within the ligament on T2-weighted coronal images. Proximal detachment or avulsion of the ligament from the lateral epicondyle may be present. With more extensive injury, complete absence of the ligament may be present, with edema and hemorrhage extending into the capsuloligamentous defect. When there is coexisting lateral epicondylitis, abnormal signal within the common extensor tendon is also present.

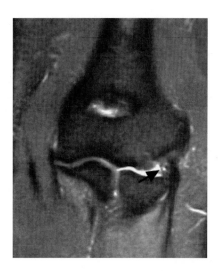

FIGURE 2.20C-2

REFERENCES

1. Daniels DL, Mallisee TA, Erickson SJ, et al. The elbow joint: osseous and ligamentous structures. *Radiographics* 1998;18:229–236.
2. Fritz RC, Steinbach LS. Magnetic resonance imaging of the musculoskeletal system: Part 3. The elbow. *Clin Orthop* 1996;Mar(324):321–339.
3. Desharnais L, Kaplan PA, Dussault RG. MR imaging of ligamentous abnormalities of the elbow. *Magn Reson Imaging Clin N Am* 1997;5:515–528.
4. Schenk M, Dalinka MK. Imaging of the elbow. An update. *Orthop Clin North Am* 1997;28:517–535.
5. Horton MG, Timins ME. MR imaging of injuries to the small joints. *Radiol Clin North Am* 1997;35:671–700.

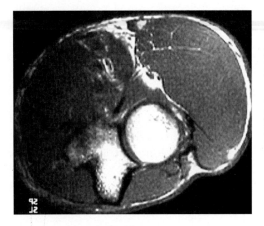

FIGURE 2.21A

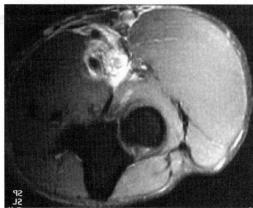

FIGURE 2.21B

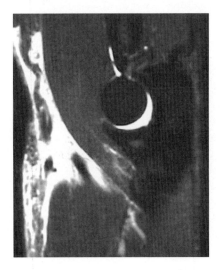

FIGURE 2.21C

CLINICAL HISTORY

A 35-year-old weightlifter felt a sudden pop while lifting his garage door.

FINDINGS

The axial T1-weighted image of the elbow obtained at the level of the radial head shows an irregular region of intermediate signal intensity in the expected position of the distal biceps tendon (Fig. 2.21A). The axial fat-suppressed proton-density-weighted image shows increased signal at the same area (Fig. 2.21B). The normal low-signal tendon is absent on both axial images. The sagittal STIR image demonstrates complete disruption of the distal biceps tendon. The tendon end is retracted proximally and has a wavy contour (Fig. 2.21C). There is edema and fluid tracking proximally along the course of the torn tendon. Soft-tissue edema is present anterior to the elbow joint.

DIAGNOSIS

Rupture of the distal biceps tendon with retraction of the torn tendon.

DISCUSSION

Rupture of the distal biceps brachii tendon is relatively uncommon, accounting for approximately 3% of all biceps injuries (1,2). Distal bicipital tendon rupture most commonly develops in middle-aged males and affects the dominant arm in more than 80% of cases (1). Body builders, weightlifters, and manual laborers tend to develop rupture of the bicipital tendon at a younger age, presumably due to repetitive injury of the tendon. Concomitant use of anabolic steroids significantly increases the likelihood of developing a spontaneous rupture of the tendon (3,4). Signs and symptoms of bicipital tendon rupture include pain and swelling in the antecubital fossa and weakness of elbow flexion and forearm supination.

The biceps brachii muscle lies within the anterior compartment of the elbow, superficial to the brachialis muscle. The biceps function in conjunction with the brachialis to flex the elbow and supinate the forearm. The biceps brachii has two heads proximally. The long head arises from the supraglenoid tubercle and superior glenoid labrum, whereas the short head arises from the coracoid process of the scapula. The biceps descend anterior to the brachialis muscle and tendon and then curve laterally to insert onto the bicipital tuberosity of the radius just distal to the elbow joint. At its distal attachment, the biceps brachii has a single tendon surrounded by a synovial tendon sheath. A small bicipital radial bursa separates the tendon from the radial tuberosity just proximal to the tendon insertion (4). The distal tendon has an aponeurotic attachment, known as the lacertus fibrosus, that extends from the myotendinous junction of the tendon to the medial deep fascia of the forearm. The median nerve and brachial artery medial to the distal biceps tendon are covered by the lacertus fibrosus. When the biceps tendon is ruptured, the lacertus fibrosus may also be torn, allowing the tendon to retract proximally. The proximally retracted tendon and muscle produce a palpable mass anteriorly at the middle upper arm, often termed the *Popeye deformity* (2). When the lacertus fibrosus is intact, the diagnosis of biceps tendon tear is more difficult, as the tendon is unable to retract significantly (4).

The distal tendon has a hypovascular zone in its distal portion that can be impinged between the ulna and the radius during pronation. This avascular zone is predisposed to develop degenerative changes, which weaken the tendon at or near its insertion site. A complete rupture of the biceps tendon at its hypovascular zone is more common than the development of partial tears. Distal biceps tendon rupture is usually an acute event that takes place following a minor injury in the setting of an underlying degenerated tendon. The typical mechanism of injury is sudden contraction of the biceps against resistance while the elbow is in moderate flexion (2,5,6).

MR imaging is useful for preoperative planning or to establish the diagnosis of distal biceps tendon rupture in those patients with an equivocal physical examination. MR imaging clearly delineates the degree of the tendon injury, the location of the tendon abnormality, and the amount of retraction present in those patients with a completely torn tendon. Tendinosis shows diffusely increased signal intensity in the tendon on T1-weighted images without increased signal intensity on the T2-weighted images. A large amount of fluid in the tendon sheath may be present in patients with tenosynovitis and the tendon may appear thickened and irregular. A partial tear of the tendon is characterized by intratendinous fluid signal intensity within the distal portion of the tendon as well as fluid around the tendon. Tendon thinning or tendon enlargement can be observed but the tendon remains continuous. A complete tendon tear is characterized by absence or discontinuity of the low-signal-intensity tendon near its insertion site. Owing to the oblique orientation of the tendon, the tear of the tendon is best seen on a combination of axial and sagittal images. The presence of a gap in the tendon is diagnostic of a complete tendon rupture. This gap can be seen on both the sagittal and axial images, but the axial images are more specific for identifying a complete absence of fiber continuity. With complete rupture, the distal T2-weighted axial images show an empty tendon sheath that contains no tendon and is instead filled with fluid or hematoma. The degree of retraction of the tendon is best determined on the sagittal images. In more chronic tears, atrophy of the biceps muscle may be present (1,5).

REFERENCES

1. Fitzgerald SW, Curry DR, Erickson SJ, et al. Distal biceps tendon injury: MR imaging diagnosis. *Radiology* 1994;191:203–206.
2. Logan PM, Janzen DL, Connell DG. Tear of the distal biceps tendon presenting as an antecubital mass: magnetic resonance imaging appearances. *Can Assoc Radiol J* 1996;47:342–346.
3. Schenk M, Dalinka MK. Imaging of the elbow. An update. *Orthop Clin North Am* 1997;28:517–535.
4. Fritz RC. MR imaging of sports injuries of the elbow. *Magn Reson Imaging Clin N Am* 1999;7:51–72.
5. Falchook FS, Zlatkin MB, Erbacher GE, et al. Rupture of the distal biceps tendon: evaluation with MR imaging. *Radiology* 1994;190:659–663.
6. Fritz RC, Steinbach LS. Magnetic resonance imaging of the musculoskeletal system: Part 3. The elbow. *Clin Orthop* 1996;Mar(324):321–339.

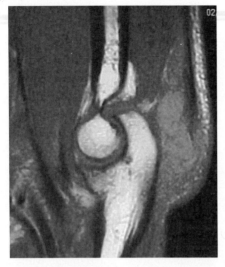

FIGURE 2.22A

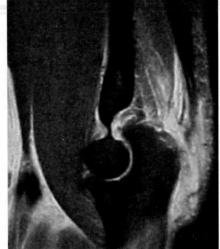

FIGURE 2.22B

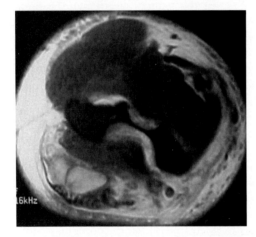

FIGURE 2.22C

CLINICAL HISTORY

This 22-year-old man sustained a sports-related injury.

FINDINGS

On the sagittal T1-weighted image of the elbow, a large high-signal hematoma surrounds the insertion site of the triceps tendon on the olecranon process of the ulna (Fig. 2.22A). The STIR sagittal image (Fig. 2.22B) shows extensive increased signal in the soft tissues in the corresponding region. The low-signal triceps tendon (Fig. 2.22A–B) is no longer attached to the olecranon. Edema is present within the deep fibers of the distal triceps muscle, which is also torn (Fig. 2.22A–B). The axial proton-density-weighted sequence (Fig. 2.22C) shows that the disrupted tendon is displaced posteriorly by the large hematoma.

DIAGNOSIS

Rupture of the distal triceps tendon with associated hematoma.

DISCUSSION

The triceps muscle lies posterior to the humerus. The triceps muscle and the much smaller anconeus muscle form the posterior compartment of the elbow (1). The triceps muscle has three proximal heads. The long head arises from the infraglenoid tubercle of the scapula. The second head, referred to as the lateral head, arises from the proximal posterolateral humeral shaft. The third head, known as the medial head, arises more distally from the posteromedial humerus (2). The distal tendon begins to form at the mid-level of the muscle, with the tendon forming in the superficial portions of the muscle. The triceps tendon, together with the deeper muscle fibers of the triceps, inserts on the posterior superior surface of the olecranon (3).

Tears of the distal triceps tendon are one of the least common tendon injuries in the body (3). Fewer than 100 cases have been reported in the literature (2,4). The typical mechanism of injury is forceful elbow flexion against the resistance of a contracting triceps muscle, as occurs during a fall on an outstretched arm. A direct blow to the posterior elbow is a less common mechanism for triceps tendon rupture (2). Systemic conditions such as anabolic steroid ingestion, chronic renal failure, hyperparathyroidism, rheumatoid arthritis, and systemic lupus erythematosus increase the risk of spontaneous rupture of the triceps tendon (5,6).

Partial tears of the triceps tendon can be managed conservatively (6). Unfortunately, complete rupture of the tendon at its insertion is much more common than a partial tear. A small avulsion fracture of the olecranon is present in approximately 80% of patients with complete rupture (2). The most common location is at or immediately adjacent to its insertion site. Development of a proximal tear at the myotendinous junction is rare (2). Clinically, patients experience the acute onset of focal pain and swelling. Following a complete rupture of the tendon, a focal defect may be palpated posterior to the elbow and the patient is unable to actively extend the elbow (6). The treatment of a complete tear of the triceps tendon is immediate surgical reattachment of the triceps tendon. Missed diagnosis or delayed repair leads to severe functional impairment.

Like the biceps tendon, the triceps tendon is best evaluated in the sagittal and axial planes. The low-signal band of the normal triceps tendon typically appears lax and redundant when the elbow is fully extended. This waviness of the tendon in the extended position, which is the normal position of the elbow during routine MR imaging, should not be interpreted as abnormal. When the tendon is redundant, the magic angle artifact can cause multiple areas of increased signal within the tendon on short TE sequences that disappear on the T2-weighted images.

Partial tears of the triceps tendon usually involve the central third of the tendon adjacent to the olecranon. Focal increased signal intensity is present on both the T1- and T2-weighted sequences and the tendon may appear thickened. In a complete tear of the tendon, no fibers of the superficial tendon attach to the bone. In patients with complete rupture of the tendon, the deeper muscular portions of the triceps muscle may still remain attached to the olecranon (2). The degree of retraction of the tendon is maximal when the deep muscular attachment is also torn. Retraction is easiest to appreciate when the elbow is flexed, allowing maximal separation between the torn tendon margins. T2-weighted and STIR sequences are best for visualization of the tear and the surrounding edema. Fluid within the olecranon bursa overlying the injured tendon, as well as an effusion within the underlying elbow joint, is present in patients with acute triceps tendon injury (2,4). Edema of the olecranon is common if there is an osseous avulsion fracture, though the small bony fragment itself may be difficult to identify on the MR examination.

REFERENCES

1. Schenk M, Dalinka MK. Imaging of the elbow. An update. *Orthop Clin North Am* 1997;28:517–535.
2. Fritz RC. MR imaging of sports injuries of the elbow. *Magn Reson Imaging Clin N Am* 1999;7:51–72.
3. Ho CP. Sports and occupational injuries of the elbow: MR imaging findings. *AJR* 1995;164:1465–1471.
4. Fritz RC, Stoller DW. The elbow. In: Stoller DW, ed. *Magnetic resonance imaging in orthopedics and sports medicine,* 2nd ed. Philadelphia: Lippincott-Raven, 1996:Chapter 10.
5. Horton MG, Timins ME. MR imaging of injuries to the small joints. *Radiol Clin North Am* 1997;35:671–700.
6. Resnick D, Kang HS. Elbow. In: Resnick D, Kang HS, eds. *Internal derangements of joints.* Philadelphia: WB Saunders, 1997:359–364.

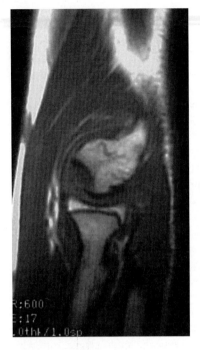

FIGURE 2.23A

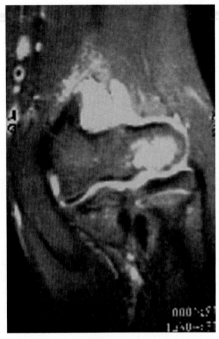

FIGURE 2.23B

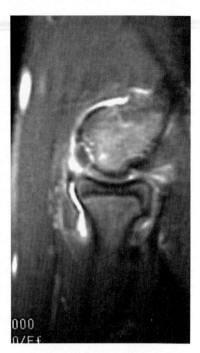

FIGURE 2.23C

CLINICAL HISTORY

A 15-year-old boy complained of 6 months of mild elbow pain.

FINDINGS

The sagittal T1-weighted image shows a concave defect involving the anterior surface of the capitellum of the humerus (Fig. 2.23A). Low signal intensity of bony fragment fills the defect. The coronal fat-suppressed proton density through the same area shows increased signal (Fig. 2.23B). A curvilinear high signal, suggesting fluid or granu-lation tissue, between the bony fragments and the parent capitellum is evident on sagittal fat-suppressed proton density (Fig. 2.23C). Underlying cartilage defect is also present. There is a moderate amount of joint fluid. The radius is normal.

DIAGNOSIS

Osteochondritis dissecans of the capitellum.

DISCUSSION

The capitellum is a semicircular prominence arising from the anterolateral portion of the distal humeral. It forms a significant portion of the lateral humeral condyle as it articulates with the proximal head of the radius. The capitelloradial articulation participates in flexion and extension at the elbow joint. The capitelloradial joint is also involved in forearm pronation and supination, as the radius rotates around the relatively fixed ulna. In the elbow, the capitellum is the most common site of osteochondritis dissecans. Osteochondritis dissecans typically develops in the anterior portion of the capitellar articular surface. The typical age of presentation is during adolescence, with the peak age between 13 and 16 years. The dominant arm of baseball players or gymnasts is more commonly involved (1).

Osteochondritis dissecans is a pathologic process in which there is a partial or total separation of a fragment of subchondral bone from the remainder of the articulating surface (1). The fragment of bone typically remains attached to its overlying cartilage. The cartilage overlying the lesion may also be isolated from the remainder of the articular cartilage, or it may maintain continuity with the adjacent cartilage, thereby stabilizing the underlying fragment of bone. Stable lesions of osteochondritis dissecans remain *in situ* and may heal spontaneously. Unstable fragments with disrupted overlying cartilage may also remain *in situ* for some time. Ultimately, loose fragments completely detach from the parent bone and migrate away from the parent site into the joint, forming a loose intraarticular body (2). The etiology of osteochondritis dissecans is not completely understood. It has been suggested that repetitive microtrauma from chronic lateral impaction of the elbow causes focal arterial injury to the capitellum, leading to osteonecrosis of a fragment of the subchondral bone (3–5). If untreated, osteochondritis dissecans of the capitellum leads to osteoarthritis of the elbow in more than 50% of patients at long-term follow-up (6). If the fragment is stable, treatment is usually conservative. If MR demonstrates the presence of an unstable fragment, surgical debridement is suggested (3).

MR imaging provides useful information in patients with osteochondritis dissecans that aids in determining optimal therapy. MR can evaluate the viability of the bone fragment, the signal characteristics of the interface of the fragment with the parent bone, and the status of the overlying cartilage; it can also identify large intraarticular bodies (1,7,8). All three image planes should be obtained. The signal within the bone fragment is diminished on the T1-weighted sequence if the area of osteochondritis dissecans is necrotic. The interface between the bone fragment and the adjacent bone should be carefully evaluated on the T2-weighted sequences. Increased signal intensity at the interface between the fragment and the parent bone can be due to the presence of intravasated joint fluid or granulation tissue at the interface. In either case, presence of a prominent high-signal interface indicates that the fragment is generally unstable and no longer contiguous with the underlying bone. The status of the overlying cartilage is an important prognostic feature in osteochondritis dissecans. Cartilage disruption implies instability and allows joint fluid to enter the interface, inhibiting the potential for healing of the fragment. Evaluation of the thin cartilage overlying the capitellum is difficult unless there is a large effusion within the elbow joint. Intraarticular injection of gadolinium followed by MR imaging improves the ability of the examination to assess the integrity of the cartilage in patients with osteochondritis dissecans (7). Intravasation of gadolinium between the fragment and the underlying bone is diagnostic of a separated fragment and disruption of the overlying articular cartilage.

REFERENCES

1. Schenk M, Dalinka MK. Imaging of the elbow. An update. *Orthop Clin North Am* 1997;28:517–535.
2. Fritz RC, Steinbach LS. Magnetic resonance imaging of the musculoskeletal system: Part 3. The elbow. *Clin Orthop* 1996;Mar(324):321–339.
3. Field LD, Savoie FH. Common elbow injuries in sport. *Sports Med* 1998;26:193–205.
4. Clanton TO, DeLee JC. Osteochondritis dissecans: history, pathophysiology and current treatment concepts. *Clin Orthop* 1982;July(167):50–64.
5. Langer F, Percy EC. Osteochondritis dissecans and anomalous centres of ossification: a review of 80 lesions in 61 patients. *Can J Surg* 1971;14:208–215.
6. Fritz RC. MR imaging of sports injuries of the elbow. *Magn Reson Imaging Clin N Am* 1999;7:51–72.
7. Resnick D, Kang HS. Elbow. In: Resnick D, Kang HS, eds. *Internal derangements of joints.* Philadelphia: WB Saunders, 1997:370–373.
8. Takahara M, Shundo M, Kondo M, et al. Early detection of osteochondritis dissecans of the capitellum in young baseball players. Report of three cases. *J Bone Joint Surg [Am]* 1998;80:892–897.

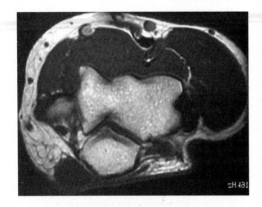

FIGURE 2.24A

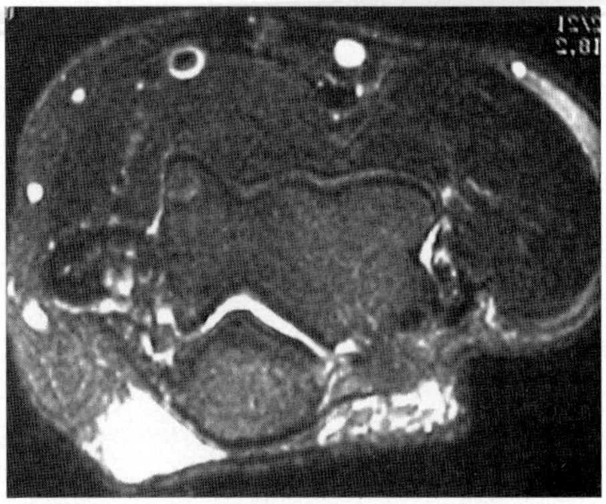

FIGURE 2.24B

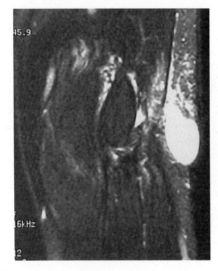

FIGURE 2.24C

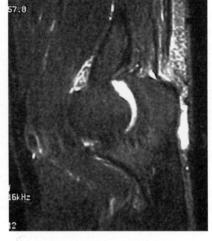

FIGURE 2.24D

CLINICAL HISTORY

A 64-year-old man with elbow pain and swelling.

FINDINGS

The axial T1-weighted image through the elbow demonstrates a well-circumscribed, homogeneous, low-signal-intensity mass (Fig. 2.24A) in the subcutaneous tissue posteromedial to the olecranon process. On the axial (Fig. 2.24B) and sagittal (Fig. 2.24C) fat-suppressed T2-weighted images, this mass shows homogeneous high signal intensity (Fig. 2.24B–C) consistent with a fluid collection. Subcutaneous edema is present around the fluid collection. Edema is also seen within the medial aspect of the distal triceps muscle (Fig. 2.24C). The distal triceps tendon is partially torn (Fig. 2.24D).

DIAGNOSIS

Olecranon bursitis associated with a partial tear of the distal triceps tendon.

DISCUSSION

The numerous normally occurring paraarticular fluid collections present in the body are generally divided into deep or superficial bursae. The deep bursae are present at birth, whereas the superficial bursae develop later in life (1). Many of these bursal fluid collections are located in the superficial joints, where they serve to minimize friction over bony prominences. In the region of the olecranon process, the normally occurring bursae include the deep subtendinous bursa and intratriceps tendon bursa, as well as numerous superficial bursae that overlie the olecranon. The most common clinically symptomatic bursitis in the elbow regions involves the subcutaneous bursa that lies posteromedial to the olecranon process (1). Symptomatic bursitis is caused by a combination of synovial inflammation and fluid accumulation within the bursa.

Inflammation of the subcutaneous olecranon bursa has been termed *miner's elbow* or *dialysis elbow* (2,3). It is most commonly caused by acute trauma or chronic repetitive overuse or pressure over this region. Olecranon bursitis is common in athletes who play football, play ice hockey, or are involved in wrestling. Association of subcutaneous olecranon bursitis with tendinosis or tears of the triceps tendon is well recognized (1). Olecranon bursitis is also commonly seen in patients who have systemic diseases such as rheumatoid arthritis, gout and other crystal deposition diseases, and chronic hemodialysis (4).

In 80% of patients with olecranon bursitis, the inflammatory changes within the synovium are due to mechanical injury, systemic arthritis, or crystal deposition. However, 20% of patients who develop acute bursitis actually have a septic bursitis, a much more serious disorder that requires aggressive antibiotic therapy or debridement (1). The most common organism responsible for bursal infection is *Staphylococcus aureus*, followed by *Streptococcus pneumoniae* and other streptococci. Septic bursitis is typically caused by penetrating trauma to the soft tissues overlying the bony prominence of the olecranon; less commonly, it is due to hematogenous spread. Infection of the olecranon bursa is more common in men than in women, presumably because of their higher risk for penetrating trauma (3).

The MR appearance of olecranon bursitis varies, depending on the severity and chronicity of the bursitis (4). Bland mechanical bursitis is characterized by the accumulation of a well-defined collection of homogeneous fluid that is low signal on the T1-weighted sequences and increases in signal with T2 weighting. Large amounts of fluid can accumulate within the bursa, but the collection remains separate from the elbow articulation as long as the triceps tendon is intact. Hemorrhage due to synovial injury may be present in the bursa, resulting in more complicated signal characteristics, depending on the age of the blood. Chronic bursitis results in septation within the mass, and an admixture of different fluids and fibrosis within the mass causes it to appear as a complex lesion. Chronic gouty bursitis often has a very complex appearance, with an admixture of high-signal fluid and low-signal deposits of urate in the bursa. It is difficult to distinguish chronic bursitis and gouty bursitis from a solid mass, even following the administration of intravenous contrast material. In synovial inflammatory diseases, particularly rheumatoid arthritis and septic bursitis, the synovial lining may be prominently thickened and enhance avidly with gadolinium. In rheumatoid arthritis, fibrous nodules can stud the synovium and multiple rice bodies may be seen within the joint. Bursitis associated with triceps tendon pathology is readily diagnosed by noting the presence of a tear of the triceps. Complete tears of the triceps allow communication of the bursa with the elbow articulation so a prominent effusion within the joint can be seen in such patients.

REFERENCES

1. Fritz RC, Stoller DW. The elbow. In: Stoller DW, ed. *Magnetic resonance imaging in orthopedics and sports medicine*, 2nd ed. Philadelphia: Lippincott-Raven, 1996:Chapter 10.
2. Resnick D, Niwayama G. Parathyroid disorders and renal osteodystrophy. In: Resnick D, Niwayama G, eds. *Diagnosis of bone and joint disorders*, 3rd ed. Philadelphia: WB Saunders, 1996:Chapter 57.
3. Resnick D, Niwayama G. Osteomyelitis, septic arthritis and soft tissue infection: mechanisms and situations. In: Resnick D, Niwayama G, eds. *Diagnosis of bone and joint disorders*, 3rd ed. Philadelphia: WB Saunders, 1996:Chapter 64.
4. Resnick D, Kang HS. Elbow. In: Resnick D, Kang HS, eds. *Internal derangements of joints*. Philadelphia: WB Saunders, 1997:376–379.

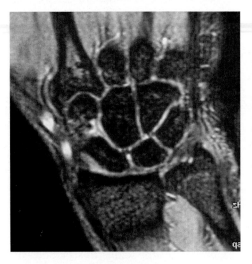

FIGURE 3.25A

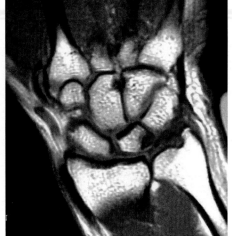

FIGURE 3.25B

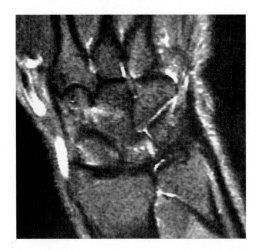

FIGURE 3.25C

CLINICAL HISTORY

A 49-year-old woman with chronic ulnar-sided wrist pain.

FINDINGS

Coronal gradient-echo (Fig. 3.25A) and T1-weighted (Fig. 3.25B) images of the wrist demonstrate deformity of the triangular fibrocartilage. Abnormal increased signal intensity is noted within the radial and middle portions of the triangular fibrocartilage. The coronal short tau inversion recovery (STIR) image shows fluid signal within the same area (Fig. 3.25C). The inferomedial lunate also shows signal abnormalities, with regions of abnormal low signal on the T1-weighted image (Fig. 3.25B) and high signal on the STIR-weighted image (Fig. 3.25C), consistent with marrow edema. The ulna is in neutral position with respect to the radius.

DIAGNOSIS

Tear of the triangular fibrocartilage with ulnar impaction syndrome.

DISCUSSION

The triangular fibrocartilage complex is composed of the triangular fibrocartilage, the dorsal and volar radioulnar ligaments, the ulnomeniscal homolog, the ulnar collateral ligament, and the sheath of the extensor carpi ulnaris tendon. The normal triangular fibrocartilage is a biconcave band of homogeneous low signal intensity extending from the medial margin of the radius to the base of the ulnar styloid, separating the distal ulna from the proximal row of carpal bones. The fibrocartilage is triangular. Its thickened margins are referred to as the dorsal and volar radioulnar ligaments. The distal triangular fibrocartilage joins the ulnar collateral ligament to form the meniscus homolog, which inserts onto the lunate, triquetrum, hamate, and base of the fifth metacarpal (1,2). The triangular fibrocartilage complex is the major stabilizer of the distal radioulnar joint and acts as a cushion, absorbing 20% of the axial load across the radiocarpal joint (3–5).

Injury or degeneration of one or more components of the triangular fibrocartilage complex produces variable symptomatology. The most common symptoms are swelling and dorsal ulnar-sided wrist pain, with or without clicking sensation. When the ligaments are injured, instability of the distal radioulnar joint may ensue.

Diagnosis of lesions of the triangular fibrocartilage by arthrography is well documented. Conventional MR imaging and MR arthrography both have a role in the evaluation of lesions of the triangular fibrocartilage, demonstrating accuracy levels comparable to arthrography (1). On MR imaging, the normal triangular fibrocartilage appears as a homogeneously low-signal-intensity structure on all MR pulse sequences. On the coronal plane, which is the optimal plane for evaluating this structure, the triangular fibrocartilage appears as a biconcave disk. The triangular fibrocartilage often appears bifurcated at its ulnar attachment. On the sagittal plane, the triangular fibrocartilage appears discoid, with thickening at its volar and dorsal sides, owing to the formation of the dorsal and volar radioulnar ligaments. On the axial images, the triangular fibrocartilage is an equilateral triangle, with its apex attaching to the ulnar styloid and its base abutting the superior margin of the distal radial sigmoid notch of the radius.

Tears of the triangular fibrocartilage are best seen on the coronal images, followed by images obtained in the sagittal plane. On T1-weighted sequences, a tear of the triangular fibrocartilage shows increased signal intensity within the low-signal disk. Perforation of the central portion of the triangular fibrocartilage is the most common manifestation of a tear. With tears more extensive than a simple perforation, the homogeneous disk appears discontinued and fragmented, and its contour may be irregular. Variable signal characteristics are seen on the T2-weighted images, depending partially on the type of tear. Degenerative tears of the triangular fibrocartilage often show decreased signal on T2 images, whereas traumatic tears show increased signal (1,5,6). In addition, traumatic tears usually occur at the radial insertion site, whereas degenerative tears occur in the central thin part of the disk.

The presence of an ulnar plus or ulnar minus variant alters the biomechanical forces transmitted through the triangular fibrocartilage complex, leading to an increased risk of injury of the complex (1,7). In ulnar impaction syndrome, the ulna is typically long with respect to the radius, although it can occasionally be of normal length, as seen in this case. The ulnar impaction syndrome describes the soft-tissue and osseous changes resulting from chronic impaction of the distal ulna against the triangular fibrocartilage complex and ulnar-sided carpal bones. With prolonged impaction, progressive degeneration and tears of the triangular fibrocartilage develop. In addition, changes of chondromalacia develop within the lunate, triquetrum, and the head of the ulna.

REFERENCES

1. Resnick D, Kang HS. Wrist and hand. In: Resnick D, Kang HS, eds. *Internal derangements of joints.* Philadelphia: WB Saunders, 1997:408–417.
2. Golimbu CN, Firooznia H, Melone CP Jr, et al. Tears of the triangular fibrocartilage of the wrist: MR imaging. *Radiology* 1989;173:731–755.
3. Pederzini L, Luchetti R, Soragni O, et al. Evaluation of the triangular fibrocartilage complex tears by arthroscopy, arthrography, and magnetic resonance imaging. *Arthroscopy* 1992;8:191–197.
4. Yu JS. Magnetic resonance imaging of the wrist. *Orthopedics* 1994;17:1041–1048.
5. Siegel S, White LM, Brahme S. Magnetic resonance imaging of the musculoskeletal system: Part 5. The wrist. *Clin Orthop* 1996;Nov(332):281–300.
6. Stoller DW, Brody GA. The wrist and hand. In: Stoller DW, ed. *Magnetic resonance imaging in orthopedics and sports medicine,* 2nd ed. Philadelphia: Lippincott-Raven, 1996:Chapter 11.
7. Minami A, Kato H. Ulnar shortening for triangular fibrocartilage complex tears associated with ulnar positive variance. *J Hand Surg [Am]* 1998;23:904–908.

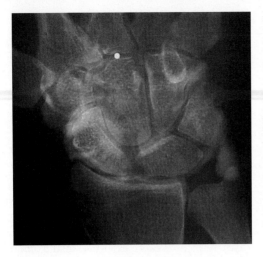

FIGURE 3.26A

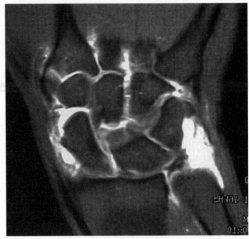

FIGURE 3.26B

CLINICAL HISTORY

A middle-aged man with ulnar-sided wrist pain.

FINDINGS

The frontal view of a wrist arthrogram was obtained following a mixed injection of iodinated contrast and diluted gadolinium into the radiocarpal joint (Fig. 3.26A). The scapholunate space is widened and contrast extends from the radiocarpal joint into the midcarpal joint via the scapholunate space. There is no contrast extravasation into the triangular fibrocartilage or into the radioulnar joint to suggest a tear of the triangular fibrocartilage. The fat-suppressed T1-weighted coronal MR image obtained following the wrist arthrogram (Fig. 3.26B) demonstrates contrast extension from the radiocarpal joint into the radioulnar joint through the radial portion of the triangular fibrocartilage. Contrast material is present throughout the wrist, with extension from the radiocarpal joint into both the midcarpal and radioulnar articulations. The scapholunate ligament is not visualized. The osseous structures are normal.

DIAGNOSIS

Tear of the triangular fibrocartilage and scapholunate ligament.

DISCUSSION

Various imaging modalities such as conventional radiography, fluoroscopy, arthrography, and MR imaging have been used for the diagnosis of the painful or unstable wrist. Diagnosis of lesions of the triangular fibrocartilage, scapholunate ligament, and lunotriquetral ligament by arthrography is well documented (1). A torn scapholunate ligament or lunotriquetral ligament allows extension of contrast from the radiocarpal joint into the midcarpal joint (1). False-negative examinations due to one-way valves can occur in this location. Therefore midcarpal injection is typically performed if the radiocarpal injection is negative. On arthrography, perforations or tears of the triangular fibrocartilage allow communication between the radiocarpal and the distal radioulnar joints. If the radiocarpal joint is injected, contrast extravasation into the distal radioulnar joint is diagnostic of a tear or perforation of the triangular fibrocartilage. Occasionally, because of a one-way valve mechanism at the tear, contrast does not extend into the radioulnar joint and a tear of the triangular fibrocartilage may remain undetected. A second injection of contrast, directly into the radioulnar joint, may identify such a tear as contrast extends into the radiocarpal joint through the torn triangular fibrocartilage.

On MR imaging, several protocols have been employed for evaluation of the triangular fibrocartilage and the intrinsic ligaments. Because of the small size of these structures, very-thin-section volume-acquisition gradient-echo sequences are very useful for assessment of the wrist. The accuracy of MR imaging for lesions of the triangular cartilage is acceptable, but assessment of the intrinsic ligaments remains problematic, with variable accuracy rates reported in the literature (2).

The normal triangular fibrocartilage is a low-signal disk of tissue that covers the distal articular surface of the ulna, separating the ulna from the overlying lunate and triquetrum. It has a broad intermediate signal attachment to the ulnar styloid and a thin attachment to the ulnar aspect of the radius. Tears of the triangular fibrocartilage show increased signal intensity within the normal low-signal disk. More extensive tears result in a discontinuous and fragmented disk. Variable signal characteristics are seen on the T2-weighted images, depending on the type of the tear. Degenerative tears of the triangular fibrocartilage often show decreased signal on T2 images, whereas traumatic tears show increased signal (1,3). Tears occur most commonly near the radial attachment of the triangular fibrocartilage. There is a normal thin extension of radial cartilage over the lip of the distal radius that underlies the meniscal attachment. This normal cartilage should not be mistaken for a tear.

MR arthrography has been proposed as a more sensitive method for diagnosis of tears of the triangular fibrocartilage. It is thought that MR arthrography is slightly more accurate than conventional MR imaging, particularly for small tears or perforations (4). In the presence of articular contrast, the triangular fibrocartilage, intrinsic ligaments, and articular surfaces are better outlined (5). Contrast filling the midcarpal or distal radioulnar joint after injection of the radiocarpal joint is diagnostic of a communicating defect in one of the intrinsic ligaments or the triangular fibrocartilage, respectively.

REFERENCES

1. Resnick D, Kang HS. Wrist and hand. In: Resnick D, Kang HS, eds. *Internal derangements of joints.* Philadelphia: WB Saunders, 1997:400–407.
2. Brown RR, Fliszar E, Cotten A, et al. Extrinsic and intrinsic ligaments of the wrist: normal and pathologic anatomy at MR arthrography with three-compartment enhancement. *Radiographics* 1998;18:667–674.
3. Siegel S, White LM, Brahme S. Magnetic resonance imaging of the musculoskeletal system: Part 5. The wrist. *Clin Orthop* 1996;Nov(332):281–300.
4. Oneson SR, Scales LM, Erickson SJ, et al. MR imaging of the painful wrist. *Radiographics* 1996;16:997–1008.
5. Beaulieu CF, Ladd AL. MR arthrography of the wrist: scanning-room injection of the radiocarpal joint based on clinical landmarks. *AJR* 1998;170:606–608.

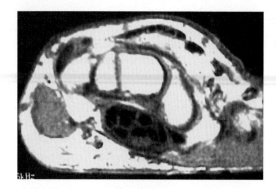

FIGURE 3.27A

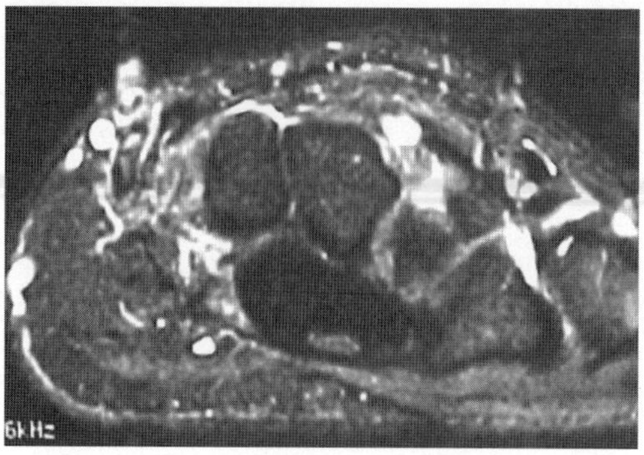

FIGURE 3.27B

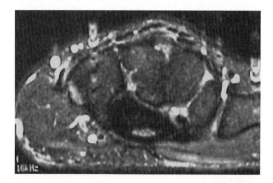

FIGURE 3.27C

CLINICAL HISTORY

This middle-aged woman complained of pain and numbness in the volar aspect of the wrist that worsened at night.

FINDINGS

On the axial T1-weighted image through the proximal wrist (Fig. 3.27A), the median nerve is enlarged, with a diameter greater than that of the adjacent flexor tendons. Within the proximal carpal tunnel, the median nerve becomes flattened and its signal intensity is increased on this axial fat-suppressed T2-weighted image (Fig. 3.27B). Further distally, at the level of the hook of the hamate, the median nerve is even more flattened and has very high signal intensity (Fig. 3.27C). The flexor retinaculum appears slightly bowed on this fat-suppressed T2-weighted image.

DIAGNOSIS

Carpal tunnel syndrome.

DISCUSSION

Carpal tunnel syndrome is a chronic debilitating condition caused by compression of the median nerve at the carpal tunnel. It is the most common of the peripheral nerve entrapment syndromes. The syndrome commonly occurs between the ages of 35 and 60 and is three to five times more common in women (1,2). The symptoms usually involve the dominant hand but can be bilateral in up to 45% of cases. Symptoms are often exacerbated at night or during repetitive daily activity. Patients experience pain and paresthesias along the distribution of the median nerve, most commonly along the index finger. With more severe carpal tunnel syndrome, pain and paresthesia can extend proximally into the volar side of the forearm. Sensory loss, muscle weakness, and thenar atrophy may develop (1,2).

The carpal tunnel is a confined space on the volar aspect of the wrist articulation. Its medial, lateral, and dorsal boundaries are formed by the anterior surface of the carpal bones. The volar surface is bounded by the flexor retinaculum, a thick fibrous band that attaches medially to the pisiform and the hook of the hamate, and laterally to the tubercle of the trapezium and the scaphoid. The major structures that pass through the carpal tunnel include the eight tendons of the flexor digitorum superficialis and flexor digitorum profundus, the flexor pollicis longus tendon, the median nerve, a small amount of fat between the flexor tendons and the volar carpal ligaments, and bursae (1).

Conditions that decrease the volume or increase the pressure within the confined space of the carpal tunnel cause compression of the median nerve, leading to focal demyelination and nerve ischemia. The many causes of carpal tunnel syndrome are often divided into acute and chronic conditions. Acute carpal tunnel syndrome is uncommon. The most common acute cause of carpal tunnel syndrome is a fracture of the distal radius or a fracture and/or dislocation of the carpal bones. Chronic carpal tunnel syndrome is much more common and is typically caused by nonspecific flexor tenosynovitis. Tenosynovitis from systemic disorders such as rheumatoid arthritis, gout, calcium pyrophosphate dihydrate crystal deposition disease, chronic infection, diabetes, lupus, and congestive heart failure can also cause carpal tunnel syndrome (1). Focal-space-occupying lesions within the carpal tunnel are another important cause of chronic carpal tunnel syndrome. Such lesions include ganglion cyst, lipoma, accessory muscles, hemangioma, synovial sarcoma, neurofibroma, and fibroma (3). Less commonly, bony deformities and advanced osteoarthritis can cause narrowing of the carpal tunnel. Physiologic changes such as pregnancy, menopause, and work-related hypertrophy of muscles and tendons are other causes (3).

The diagnosis of carpal tunnel syndrome is primarily based on history and physical findings, with confirmation by electrophysiologic evaluation. Diagnostic imaging plays a minor role in evaluating carpal tunnel syndrome (1,2). MR imaging has been used to establish the diagnosis of carpal tunnel syndrome and for identification of space-occupying lesions within the carpal tunnel. The axial images are the best plane for evaluation of this region. Findings in carpal tunnel syndrome include increased size of the median nerve proximal to the carpal tunnel, secondary to hyperemia and edema. The enlargement is most prominent at the level of the pisiform. The normal median nerve is approximately the same size as the flexor tendons, which can be used for comparison. Within the carpal tunnel, the median nerve is flattened, particularly at the level of the hook of the hamate. Increased signal intensity of the median nerve due to edema on T2-weighted images is present. Volar bowing of the flexor retinaculum due to increased pressure can be seen. Bowing is best evaluated at the distal carpal tunnel between the hook of the hamate and the tubercle of the trapezium, where the flexor retinaculum is thickest and the carpal tunnel is narrowest (1,4,5). Unfortunately, these signs are nonspecific and can be seen in asymptomatic individuals. Therefore isolated findings must be correlated with the clinical examination. A combination of these findings improves the sensitivity and specificity of the MR examination, particularly the combination of high signal intensity within the median nerve and retinacular bowing (2).

Other MR findings are based on the specific etiology of the carpal tunnel syndrome. In tenosynovitis, the tendon sheath is enlarged and the tendons are separated by fluid within the tendon sheaths. A joint effusion may be present. Masses and ganglion cysts may be easily identified on the T2-weighted images. Articular diseases and other systemic causes may be delineated that help preoperative planning. MR imaging can also be employed to evaluate the postoperative wrist in patients with failed carpal tunnel release to look for fibrosis, incomplete excision of the retinaculum, residual mass effect, or other causes of failed surgery.

REFERENCES

1. Mesgarzadeh M, Triolo J, Schneck CD. Carpal tunnel syndrome: MR imaging diagnosis. *Magn Reson Imaging Clin N Am* 1995;3:249–264.
2. Radack DM, Schweitzer ME, Taras J. Carpal tunnel syndrome: Are the MR findings a result of population selection bias? *AJR* 1997;169:1649–1653.
3. Nakamichi K, Tachibana S. Unilateral carpal tunnel syndrome and space-occupying lesions. *J Hand Surg [Br]* 1993;18:748–749.
4. Seyfert S, Boegner F, Hamm B, et al. The value of magnetic resonance imaging in carpal tunnel syndrome. *J Neurol* 1994;242:41–46.
5. Mesgarzadeh M, Schneck CD, Bonakdarpour A, et al. Carpal tunnel: MR imaging: Part II. Carpal tunnel syndrome. *Radiology* 1989;171:749–754.

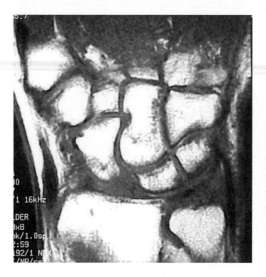

FIGURE 3.28A

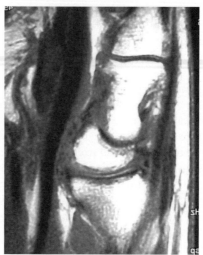

FIGURE 3.28B

CLINICAL HISTORY

A middle-aged woman complained of chronic wrist pain.

FINDINGS

The coronal T1-weighted image of the wrist (Fig. 3.28A) shows widening of the scapholunate space, amorphous signal intensity between the scaphoid and the lunate, and disruption of the interosseous ligament. The lunotriquetral ligament is intact. On the sagittal T1-weighted image through the lunate (Fig. 3.28B), the lunate is tilted dorsally with respect to the radius and the capitate. The capitate is dorsally displaced with respect to the radius.

DIAGNOSIS

Scapholunate dissociation with dorsal intercalated segmental instability (DISI).

DISCUSSION

The carpal bones are structured in two rows in the wrist and are stabilized by a number of intrinsic and extrinsic carpal ligaments. On the coronal plane, the interosseous spaces between the carpal bones are uniform. Three smooth, parallel arcs can be drawn to define the normal intercarpal relationships (1). Arc 1 follows the proximal surfaces of the scaphoid, lunate, and triquetrum. Arc 2 runs along the distal surfaces of these same bones. Arc 3 follows the proximal surfaces of the capitate and hamate. On the sagittal plane, a vertical line can be drawn through the axes of the radius, the lunate, and the capitate. The axis of the scaphoid is normally tilted volarly 30 to 60 degrees relative to this vertical axis.

Disruption of the ligaments of the wrist disturbs the normal pattern of carpal alignment and the smooth and synchronous motions necessary for proper function of the wrist, resulting in carpal instability. The ligaments of the wrist are complex and various nomenclatures and classifications have been used to describe their anatomy. In general, the ligaments are divided into two groups: the intrinsic ligaments and the extrinsic ligaments. The intrinsic ligaments arise from and insert onto the carpal bones, whereas the extrinsic ligaments interconnect the radius or the metacarpals to the carpal bones (2). The extrinsic ligaments can be divided into the strong volar ligaments, which are important stabilizers, and the relatively weak dorsal ligaments (3,4). The principal intrinsic ligaments are the scapholunate and lunotriquitrum ligaments.

Instability of the carpal bones is subdivided into many different patterns. Carpal instability is divided into nondissociated and dissociated types. Nondissociated types are less common and are the results of disruption of the extrinsic ligaments without rupture of the intrinsic ligaments. Dissociated types are much more common and are due to disruption of both the intrinsic and extrinsic ligaments. The most common forms of dissociated carpal instability are due to disruption of the scapholunate ligament, lunotriquetral ligament, or both (1).

Scapholunate dissociation occurs where there is a tear of the scapholunate ligament and the extrinsic volar radiocarpal ligaments. This abnormality may be the result of trauma, with or without lunate or perilunate dislocation, rheumatoid arthritis, or other articular disease (1). The scapholunate distance is widened in the coronal plane to greater than 4 mm. On coronal MR imaging, the scapholunate and lunotriquetral ligaments can be identified on spin-echo or gradient-echo sequences. The ligaments appear as thin or triangular bands of low signals horizontally traversing the proximal scapholunate and lunotriquetral spaces. When there is a tear, the ligament may appear elongated, look incomplete, have an abnormal course, or be completely absent. Secondary signs include presence of fluid in the scapholunate or lunotriquetral interosseous spaces and in the adjacent midcarpal joint.

Scapholunate ligament disruption subsequently leads to DISI once the volar extrinsic ligaments are disrupted by abnormal intercarpal motion. In the presence of scapholunate dissociation, the scaphoid is unable to counteract the lunate's intrinsic dorsiflexion. The lunate subsequently migrates into a more dorsiflexed position on the sagittal plane, allowing the capitate to migrate proximally. In DISI, the scaphoid is volarly flexed and the scapholunate angle is greater than 70 degrees. DISI is best evaluated on the sagittal plane where the normal coaxial alignment of the radius, lunate, and capitate can be assessed. Proper position of the wrist is critical because prone positioning or ulnar deviation causes the normal lunate to tilt dorsally, mimicking DISI (5). MR imaging is insensitive for disruption of the extrinsic volar and dorsal ligaments, but the malalignment is diagnostic of ligament insufficiency. MR arthrography has been reported to have better sensitivity and specificity than conventional MR imaging for the direct diagnosis of carpal ligament injury (6).

REFERENCES

1. Resnick D, Kang HS. Wrist and hand. In: Resnick D, Kang HS, eds. *Internal derangements of joints.* Philadelphia: WB Saunders, 1997:420–425.
2. Reicher MA, Kellerhouse LE. Carpal instability. In: Reicher MA, Kellerhouse LE, eds. *MRI of the wrist and hand.* New York: Raven Press, 1990:73–81.
3. Brown RR, Fliszar E, Cotten A, et al. Extrinsic and intrinsic ligaments of the wrist: normal and pathologic anatomy at MR arthrography with three-compartment enhancement. *Radiographics* 1998;18:667–674.
4. Oneson SR, Scales LM, Erickson SJ, et al. MR imaging of the painful wrist. *Radiographics* 1996;16:997–1008.
5. Zanetti M, Hodler J, Gilula LA. Assessment of dorsal or ventral intercalated segmental instability configurations of the wrist: reliability of sagittal MR images. *Radiology* 1998;206:339–345.
6. Siegel S, White LM, Brahme S. Magnetic resonance imaging of the musculoskeletal system: Part 5. The wrist. *Clin Orthop* 1996;Nov(332):281–300.

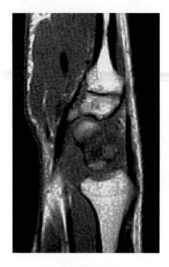

FIGURE 3.29A

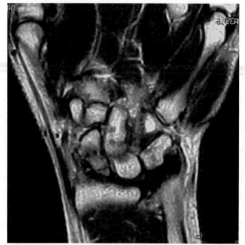

FIGURE 3.29B

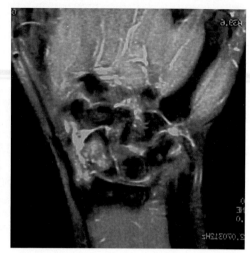

FIGURE 3.29C

CLINICAL HISTORY

A man complained of wrist pain after a fall.

FINDINGS

A sagittal T1-weighted image (Fig. 3.29A) shows amorphous low signal within the marrow of the scaphoid. In addition, several linear low-signal lines are seen traversing the waist and the proximal pole of the scaphoid. These low-signal lines persist on the T2-weighted coronal image (Fig. 3.29B). High-signal marrow edema of the scaphoid is present on the fat-suppressed proton-density image (Fig. 3.29C). The proximal pole of the scaphoid has maintained its normal shape without evidence of volume loss or fragmentation. Soft-tissue edema and a small joint effusion are present in the region of the scaphoid. The scapholunate distance is normal.

DIAGNOSIS

Comminuted scaphoid fracture.

DISCUSSION

Scaphoid fractures are the most common type of carpal fracture, representing almost three-fourths of all fractures involving the carpal bones. Scaphoid fractures predominantly occur in young active persons between the ages of 15 and 40 years, and are much less common in children and older people (1,2). These fractures are classified according to their location, which influences the rate of healing and the possibility of developing nonunion and avascular necrosis of the proximal scaphoid (3). Typical locations of fracture include the proximal pole, waist, distal body, tuberosity, and distal articular surface of the scaphoid bone. The most common site of fracture is through the waist, which is involved in about 70% of cases, followed by the proximal pole, which is fractured in about 20%. Both these types of fractures are at risk for nonunion and avascular necrosis, whereas the more distal fractures tend to heal uneventfully. The proximal fractures have a higher rate of delayed union or nonunion due to displacement of the fracture fragments, inadequate immobilization, interposition of soft tissue in the fracture site, and inadequate blood supply. The blood supply to the scaphoid enters the bone through the distal body and may be interrupted when the fracture is at the waist or proximal pole (3). Complications of scaphoid fractures are particularly common if the diagnosis is missed or delayed. These complications include delayed union, malunion, nonunion, avascular necrosis, carpal instability, and subsequent osteoarthritis within the surrounding carpal joints (1,4). Therefore imaging plays a critical role in early diagnosis of this significant injury (4).

The most common clinical symptom of a scaphoid fracture is pain in the anatomic snuffbox. Although snuffbox pain is highly sensitive for the diagnosis of scaphoid fracture, the specificity of this sign is as low as 40%. Conventional radiographs are usually obtained initially, and most scaphoid fractures can be detected. Unfortunately, undisplaced fractures can be easily overlooked on routine radiography. If there is clinical suspicion of a scaphoid fracture, patients with normal or equivocal radiographs routinely undergo wrist immobilization and follow-up radiographs in 10 to 14 days. To avoid such prolonged immobilization, bone scintigraphy and computed tomography scanning have been utilized in the acute phase to identify radiographically occult scaphoid injury (5). More recently, the role of MR imaging for occult bone trauma has been emphasized. MR imaging has shown to be very sensitive and specific in detecting acute fractures. The fracture planes and the degree of displacement or angulation of the fracture fragments can be better determined because of the multiplanar imaging capabilities of this modality. In an acute fracture, edema or hemorrhage leads to low to intermediate signal in the T1-weighted sequence around the fracture site. The area of edema shows increased signal on T2-weighted and fat-suppressed images. Linear low-signal-intensity bands that remain low signal on both T1- and T2-weighted images are consistent with a fracture line. In the presence of a scaphoid fracture, additional osseous and soft-tissue injuries can also be identified and evaluated (1,3,5).

MR imaging can also be used for evaluation of the healing process. Persistent high signal intensity in the fracture site on T2-weighted images suggests nonunion, whereas marrow continuity across the fracture line is consistent with healing. When nonunion is detected but both the proximal and distal fragments show normal marrow signal, the fracture often heals with further surgical interventions. When the proximal pole shows abnormal low signal on both T1- and T2-weighted images with collapse and fibrous replacement of the bony architecture, indicating avascular necrosis, there is little likelihood of healing of the fracture and the outcome is poor (2).

REFERENCES

1. Munk PL, Lee MJ, Logan PM, et al. Scaphoid bone waist fractures, acute and chronic: imaging with different techniques. *AJR* 1997;168:779–786.
2. Morgan WJ, Breen TF, Coumas JM, et al. Role of magnetic resonance imaging in assessing factors affecting healing in scaphoid nonunions. *Clin Orthop* 1997;336:240–246.
3. Resnick D, Kang HS. Wrist and hand. In: Resnick D, Kang HS, eds. *Internal derangements of joints.* Philadelphia: WB Saunders, 1997:428–437.
4. Hunter JC, Escobedo EM, Wilson AJ, et al. MR imaging of clinically suspected scaphoid fractures. *AJR* 1997;168:1287–1293.
5. Siegel S, White LM, Brahme S. Magnetic resonance imaging of the musculoskeletal system: Part 5. The wrist. *Clin Orthop* 1996;Nov(332):281–300.

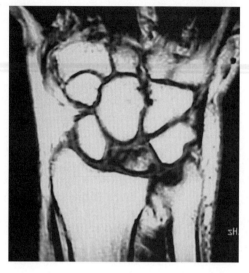

FIGURE 3.30A

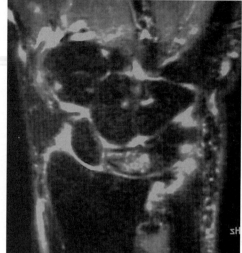

FIGURE 3.30B

CLINICAL HISTORY

A middle-aged man complained of progressive wrist pain with swelling.

FINDINGS

The coronal T1-weighted image of the wrist (Fig. 3.30A) demonstrates abnormal low signal intensity within the lunate. The superior surface of the lunate is deformed and the lunate is partially collapsed. The lunate shows patchy areas of increased signal on the coronal STIR-weighted image (Fig. 3.30B). Increased signal intensity is also noted within the radiocarpal, midcarpal, and radioulnar joints, consistent with effusion or synovitis.

DIAGNOSIS

Kienbock's disease (idiopathic osteonecrosis) of the lunate.

DISCUSSION

Osteonecrosis of the carpal bones most commonly involves the proximal scaphoid following a fracture of that bone. Idiopathic osteonecrosis of the carpal bones is most common in the lunate (Kienbock's disease), followed by the proximal scaphoid and the capitate. Osteonecrosis of the remaining carpal bones is rare (1). Kienbock's disease is relatively uncommon and appears to occur predominantly in males. It commonly occurs in young, active adults between the ages of 20 and 40, and is more common in the dominant extremity (2–4). Clinically, patients present with dorsal wrist pain and occasional soft-tissue swelling about the wrist. In advanced disease, there is decreased range of motion and decreased grip strength.

The exact etiology of osteonecrosis of the lunate is uncertain. It is believed that traumatic injury, due either to a fracture or to soft-tissue injury, causes interruption of the blood supply of the lunate. The posttraumatic devascularization of the lunate leads to osteonecrosis. Others believe that abnormal axial loading forces, especially due to the presence of ulna minus variance, subjects the lunate to increased compression or shear stresses. The third possibility is primary impairment of the lunate blood supply due to congenital or nontraumatic acquired causes (2–4).

On the basis of conventional radiographs, Kienbock's disease has been classified into five different stages, with increasing stages indicating further disease progression (2,4,5). In stage I Kienbock's disease, the lunate has a normal appearance, though microscopic fracture lines may be present. Stage II shows rarefaction of the bone along the fracture line.

In stage III disease, the lunate becomes sclerotic relative to the other carpal bones. In stage IV, the lunate loses its normal architecture and collapses due to secondary fractures. Complications as a result of lunate collapse develop in stage V, including scapholunate dissociation and secondary osteoarthritic changes of the radiocarpal joint (4,5).

MR imaging is the most sensitive and specific modality for the diagnosis of Kienbock's disease. It is superior to conventional radiographs and bone scintigraphy owing to its better space resolution and higher sensitivity for soft-tissue and bone marrow edema. The appearance of the osteonecrosis varies on MR imaging, depending on the stage of the disease. Initially, T1-weighted images show focal or diffuse low-signal-intensity areas in the necrotic marrow but the architecture of the bone is preserved. During this acute phase, the T2-weighted images show areas of intermediate or mildly increased signal, whereas the STIR images may have slightly increased signal. The increased signal intensity is initially due to hemorrhage and later due to marrow edema and the formation of granulation tissue. The low-signal areas on the T2 and STIR images probably represent regions of fibrosis. When the bone starts to collapse, initial height loss develops on the radial side of the lunate. Subsequently, the lunate collapses further from the distal to proximal direction. In the final stages of osteonecrosis, the lunate demonstrates low signal intensity on all MR sequences (1,3,6). Complications of advanced osteonecrosis, such as scapholunate dissociation and osteoarthritis of the radiocarpal joint, can also be evaluated by MR imaging.

REFERENCES

1. Resnick D, Kang HS. Wrist. In: Resnick D, Kang HS, eds. *Internal derangements of joints.* Philadelphia: WB Saunders, 1997:437–440.
2. Almquist EE. Kienbock's disease. *Clin Orthop* 1986;202:68–78.
3. Siegel S, White LM, Brahme S. Magnetic resonance imaging of the musculoskeletal system: Part 5. The wrist. *Clin Orthop* 1996;Nov(332):281–300.
4. Kellerhouse LE, Reicher MA. Osteonecrosis and fractures of the wrist. In: Reicher MA, Kellerhouse LE, eds. *MRI of the wrist and hand.* New York: Raven Press, 1990:107–111.
5. Oneson SR, Scales LM, Erickson SJ, et al. MR imaging of the painful wrist. *Radiographics* 1996;16:997–1008.
6. Stoller DW, Brody GA. The wrist and hand. In: Stoller DW, ed. *Magnetic resonance imaging in orthopedics and sports medicine,* 2nd ed. Philadelphia: Lippincott-Raven, 1996:Chapter 11.

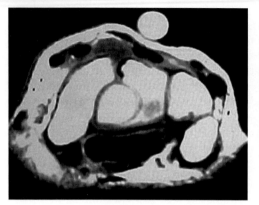

FIGURE 3.31A

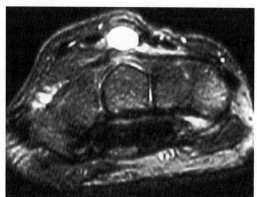

FIGURE 3.31B

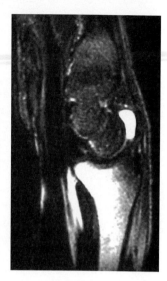

FIGURE 3.31C

CLINICAL HISTORY

A 52-year-old woman felt an enlarging mass on the dorsum of her wrist.

FINDINGS

There is a round, low-signal-intensity mass just deep to the extensor digitorum on the axial T1-weighted image (Fig. 3.31A). On the fat-suppressed T2-weighted axial (Fig. 3.31B) and sagittal (Fig. 3.31C) images, this mass shows intense homogeneous high signal intensity with a well-circumscribed border. The mass deforms and displaces the extensor digitorum tendons posteriorly. It does not appear to communicate with the radiocarpal joint. The osseous structures are normal.

DIAGNOSIS

Ganglion cyst of the dorsum of the wrist.

DISCUSSION

The ganglion cyst is the most common soft-tissue mass of the hand and wrist, representing 50% to 70% of all soft-tissue masses in this region (1–3). Ganglion cysts can develop at any age but most commonly present between the third and fifth decades, predominantly in women. Typically, a ganglion presents as a painless palpable mass. In up to 50% of cases, patients may experience vague local pain (1,3,4). Seventy percent of the ganglion cysts occur on the dorsum of the wrist, typically communicating with the scapholunate ligament. The next most common location is the volar soft tissues of the wrist, between the flexor carpi radialis and abductor pollicis longus tendons. Less common locations include the distal interphalangeal joint, the flexor retinaculum, the proximal interphalangeal joint, adjacent to an extensor tendon, the carpal tunnel, the ulnar canal, and the metacarpotrapezoid joint.

The etiology of ganglion cysts is uncertain; they are thought to be due to trauma or constant stress (3,5). The site of origin may be the joint capsule, tendon, or tendon sheath. There may be a communicating duct, especially to the scapholunate ligament (1,4,6). If arthrography or tenography is performed, a communication between the ganglion cyst and the joint can occasionally be seen. However, injection of the ganglion fails to demonstrate such communication, suggesting a one-way valve mechanism for entrapment of the joint fluid (1,3,6). The typical cyst is well defined, has a fibrous wall, and contains mucinous fluid. The cyst may contain a single cavity or be multiloculated. Most ganglion cysts are solitary, although multiple ganglion cysts can present simultaneously at the wrist. Rarely, the walls of the cyst can calcify, usually due to a complication such as internal hemorrhage. Ganglion cysts can disappear spontaneously, though they typically recur following a spontaneous rupture. They also recur in up to 50% of cases treated with cyst aspiration or sclerosis. Surgical removal of the lesion has the lowest recurrence rate.

Conventional radiographs are usually normal or show only a nonspecific soft-tissue mass. If the ganglion is adjacent to the bone, periosteal proliferation or even frank pressure erosion of the bone may be present. On MR examination, a ganglion appears as a well-defined mass that is often lobulated and contains internal septations. Typically, it measures between 1.5 and 2.5 cm in diameter. The axial plane is most helpful in identifying the lesion, although all three planes are often needed to distinguish the lesion from a joint recess (1,3,6). On T1-weighted images, the lesion is homogeneous low to intermediate signal intensity. The signal increases markedly with T2 weighting, making the lesion much easier to identify in the soft tissues. Hemorrhage into the lesion can occur, particularly following trauma to the region. In such a situation, the characteristic signal of a ganglion cyst may be altered.

REFERENCES

1. Steiner E, Steinbach LS, Schnarkowski P, et al. Ganglia and cysts around joints. *Radiol Clin North Am* 1996;34:395–425.
2. Yu JS. Magnetic resonance imaging of the wrist. *Orthopedics* 1994;17:1041–1048.
3. Steinbach LS. Tumors and synovial processes in the wrist and hand. In: Reicher MA, Kellerhouse LE, eds. *MRI of the wrist and hand.* New York: Raven Press, 1990:132–136.
4. Horton MG, Timins ME. MR imaging of injuries to the small joints. *Radiol Clin North Am* 1997;35:671–700.
5. Oneson SR, Scales LM, Erickson SJ, et al. MR imaging of the painful wrist. *Radiographics* 1996;16:997–1008.
6. Resnick D, Kang HS. Wrist and hand. In: Resnick D, Kang HS, eds. *Internal derangements of joints.* Philadelphia: WB Saunders, 1997:451–453.

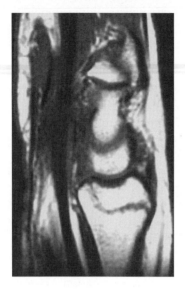
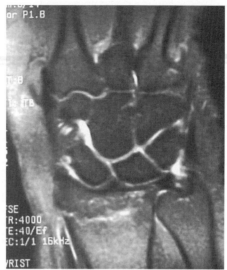

FIGURE 3.32A   **FIGURE 3.32B**

CLINICAL HISTORY

A woman had wrist pain after a fall on her outstretched hand. The radiograph of the wrist was reported to be normal.

FINDINGS

A sagittal T1-weighted image of the wrist (Fig. 3.32A) shows a horizontal linear low-signal line in the distal radial metaphysis. The linear band extends from the dorsal aspect of the radius anteriorly and distally to exit the anterosuperior articular surface. On the coronal fat-suppressed proton-density image (Fig. 3.32B), high signal intensity is noted in the same area of the distal radius. The low-signal cortex of the medial radius is disrupted. Fluid is also noted within the radiocarpal and midcarpal joints, consistent with effusion. The triangular fibrocartilage complex, articular congruence, and osseous alignment are normal.

DIAGNOSIS

Nondisplaced fracture of the distal radius.

DISCUSSION

Fractures of the distal radius are the most common fractures of the upper extremity, accounting for 17% of all fractures treated in the emergency room (1). They occur most commonly in middle-aged and elderly persons who fall on an outstretched arm (1). The distal radius is the major osseous element that supports the axial loading forces of the carpus and the radiocarpal joint. The distal radius articulates with the scaphoid, the lunate, and the ulnar head. Therefore normal alignment of the radiocarpal joint is important for the proper function of the wrist (1,2).

There are many types of distal radius fracture, and several eponyms have been used to describe the various patterns of osseous injury seen in this location. Some of the different fractures of the distal radius include the Colles', Smith's, Barton's, Hutchinson's, and die punch fractures (1,2). A Colles' fracture is a transverse fracture of the distal radius with dorsal displacement, angulation, or both. The Colles' fracture is the most common pattern of fracture of the distal radius. The less common Smith's fracture is a fracture of the distal radius with volar displacement and angulation. It is also referred to as a reverse Colles' fracture. The Barton's fracture is an oblique fracture extending to the dorsal rim of the distal radius. This fracture is unstable and is associated with subluxation of the carpus along with the displaced articular fragment. A Hutchinson's fracture involves the styloid process of the radius. The die punch fracture is a depressed central radius fracture with proximal migration of the lunate.

Diagnosis of distal radius fracture is primarily based on physical examination and conventional radiographs. Distal radius fractures are typically treated conservatively, but if there is significant angulation or step-off of the articular surface, surgical fixation is used. Improper treatment can lead to deformity of the distal radius, carpal instability, osteoarthritis, and soft-tissue and median nerve damage. MR imaging is helpful for detection of radiographically occult radial trauma, for assessment of the extent of the fracture, and for detection of the associated ligament and soft-tissue injury (2–4). MR is very sensitive in detecting bone marrow edema and occult fractures of the wrist. Occult fractures appear as linear low-signal lines in the radius on both T1- and T2-weighted images (4). The fracture line is surrounded by marrow edema, which appears as an ill-defined region of low signal intensity on T1- and high signal intensity on T2-weighted images.

MR imaging is excellent in demonstrating associated soft-tissue injuries. Tears of the triangular fibrocartilage complex (TFCC) are common in association with wrist injuries, with reported rates of 45% to 66% (3). Abnormal increased signal intensity within the homogeneous low-signal TFCC is suggestive of a tear. Disruption of the scapholunate ligament can be visualized in the presence of an intraarticular fracture of the distal radius. Other soft-tissue injuries, such as tears of the tendons or tenosynovitis, are shown on MR imaging as abnormal high signal within the tendon and fluid signal around the tendon.

REFERENCES

1. Resnick D, Goergen TG, Pathria MN. Physical injury. In: Resnick D, ed. *Bone and joint imaging.* Philadelphia: WB Saunders, 1996:769–772.
2. Kellerhouse LE, Reicher MA. Osteonecrosis and fractures of the wrist. In: Reicher MA, Kellerhouse LE, eds. *MRI of the wrist and hand.* New York: Raven Press, 1990:113–119.
3. Spence LD, Savenor A, Nwachuku I, et al. MRI of fractures of the distal radius: comparison with conventional radiographs. *Skeletal Radiol* 1998;27:244–249.
4. Metz VM, Gilula LA. Imaging techniques for distal radius fractures and related injuries. *Orthop Clin North Am* 1993;24:217–228.

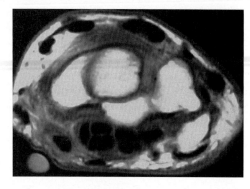

FIGURE 3.33A

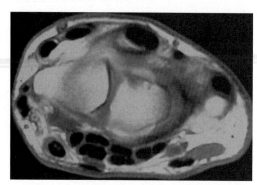

FIGURE 3.33B

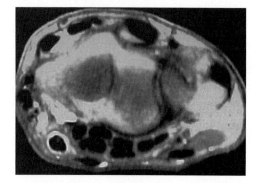

FIGURE 3.33C

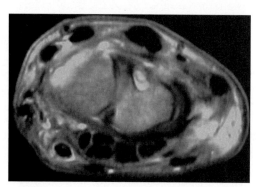

FIGURE 3.33D

CLINICAL HISTORY

A 61-year-old man with volar wrist pain and swelling.

FINDINGS

There is increased signal intensity with the flexor carpi radialis tendon on the axial T1-weighted images (Fig. 3.33A–B). The tendon is slightly enlarged and surrounded by amorphous low signal intensity. On the axial fat-suppressed proton-density-weighted images (Fig. 3.33C–D), the tendon contains small foci of increased signal intensity. The tendon is surrounded by a ring of homogeneous high signal intensity. There is a small amount of effusion within the radiocarpal joint and minor cystic changes are present within the dorsal aspect of the lunate.

DIAGNOSIS

Flexor carpi radialis tendinitis with associated tenosynovitis.

DISCUSSION

Inflammation of the flexor and extensor tendons or tendon sheaths of the wrist is common. One or multiple tendons or tendon sheaths can be affected. The inflammation may be a primary condition as part of an overuse syndrome from repetitive activity or it may be secondary to osseous abnormalities adjacent to the affected tendon, such as fractures, ganglia, osteoarthritis, and systemic inflammatory disorders (1,2). Symptoms caused by tendinitis and tenosynovitis are nonspecific, with pain and swelling being the most common complaints. Flexor carpi radialis tendinitis and tenosynovitis occur more frequently in women. Because of the location of this tendon, symptoms may mimic carpal tunnel syndrome.

The flexor carpi radialis tendon lies outside the carpal tunnel. It passes over the tubercle of the navicular bone and then under the ridge of the trapezoid to insert onto the base of the second metacarpal. The tendon has its own tendon sheath from the distal of the forearm to the distal trapezium; 90% of the space within the sheath is occupied by the tendon (1). At the level of the crest of the trapezium, the space within the tendon sheath is at its narrowest. Any condition that narrows the tendon sheath, such as fracture of the scaphoid, osteo-phytes, or a ganglion at this level, causes constriction of the tendon, resulting in tendinitis and tenosynovitis (3). In severe cases, the tendon may rupture spontaneously (4).

Since the symptoms of tendinitis and tenosynovitis are nonspecific, MR plays an important role in diagnosing this disorder. Normally, the tendon is homogeneous low signal intensity on all pulse sequences. Abnormal increased signal intensity within the tendon suggests tendinitis. When the high signal intensity extends to the surface of the tendon and fluid extends into the tendon substance, a tear is present (1,3). The involved tendon is typically thickened. The tendon sheath is distended and fluid surrounds the tendon, which is best visualized on T2-weighted images. In the chronic phase, the hyperintense signal on T2-weighted images is less striking, owing to progressive fibrosis. In the chronic phase, patients' symptoms are often worsened because of stenosis of the synovial sheath. MR is not sensitive for identifying stenosis of the sheath, but it can demonstrate thickening or rupture of the tendon in patients with chronic tendon inflammation.

REFERENCES

1. Klug JD. MR diagnosis of tenosynovitis about the wrist. *Magn Reson Imaging Clin N Am* 1995;3:305–312.
2. Gabel G, Bishop AT, Wood MB. Flexor carpi radialis tendinitis: Part II. Results of operative treatment. *J Bone Joint Surg [Am]* 1994;76:1015–1018.
3. Resnick D, Kang HS. Wrist and hand. In: Resnick D, Kang HS, eds. *Internal derangements of joints.* Philadelphia: WB Saunders, 1997:445–449.
4. Tonkin MA, Stern HS. Spontaneous rupture of the flexor carpi radialis tendon. *J Hand Surg [Br]* 1991;16:72–74.

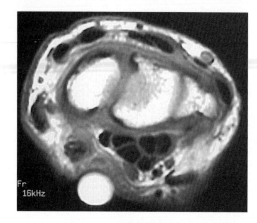

FIGURE 3.34A   **FIGURE 3.34B**

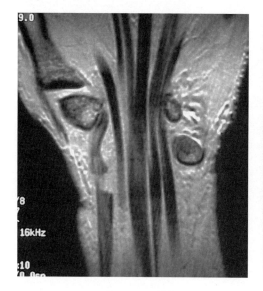

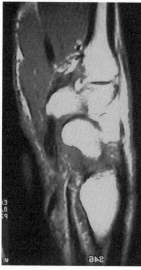

FIGURE 3.34C   **FIGURE 3.34D**

CLINICAL HISTORY

This 44-year-old woman cut her wrist with a piece of glass.

FINDINGS

On the axial T1-weighted images (Fig. 3.34A–B), abnormal signal intensity is noted within the flexor carpi radialis tendon. The tendon is deformed and appears markedly attenuated at the level of the radiocarpal joint. There is soft-tissue edema around the tendon. On the coronal gradient-echo image (Fig. 3.34C) and sagittal T1-weighted image (Fig. 3.34D), the flexor carpi radialis tendon is disrupted. The proximal portion of the tendon is retracted, leaving a 1-cm gap between the proximal and distal portions of the tendon.

DIAGNOSIS

Complete laceration of the flexor carpi radialis tendon.

DISCUSSION

Lacerations of tendons occur most frequently in the hand because of the high incidence of penetrating trauma in this region. Penetrating trauma to the volar wrist results in injury to the flexor carpi radialis tendon, which can be injured in association with vascular trauma to this region. Nontraumatic ruptures of the flexor tendons are uncommon, typically seen in association with rheumatoid arthritis or carpal osteoarthritis (1). Rupture of the tendon proximal to the carpus is uncommon in the absence of penetrating injury.

Clinical symptoms of rupture of the flexor carpi radialis tendon are often confused with carpal tunnel syndrome (1–4). MR imaging is helpful for evaluating patients with volar wrist pain and distinguishing these two entities, thereby avoiding unnecessary surgery.

MR findings of laceration of the flexor carpi radialis tendon include disruption, deformity, and discontinuity of the normal dark signal band of the tendon on both T1- and T2-weighted images. Edema or hemorrhage can be seen around the tendon and within the tendon sheath, manifest as high signal intensity on T2-weighted images. In the presence of a laceration, fluid in the soft tissues adjacent to the sheath is commonly present. Gas or foreign bodies may be detected in the soft tissues at the site of laceration. Gas and foreign bodies typically appear low signal on both the T1- and T2-weighted images.

REFERENCES

1. Tonkin MA, Stern HS. Spontaneous rupture of the flexor carpi radialis tendon. *J Hand Surg [Br]* 1991;16:72–74.
2. Klug JD. MR diagnosis of tenosynovitis about the wrist. *Magn Reson Imaging Clin N Am* 1995;3:305–312.
3. Resnick D, Kang HS. Wrist and hand. In: Resnick D, Kang HS, eds. *Internal derangements of joints.* Philadelphia: WB Saunders, 1997:445–449.
4. Reicher MA, Kellerhouse LE. Carpal tunnel disease, flexor and extensor tendon disorders. In: Reicher MA, Kellerhouse LE, eds. *MRI of the wrist and hand.* New York: Raven Press, 1990:64–67.

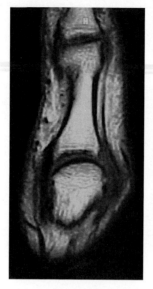 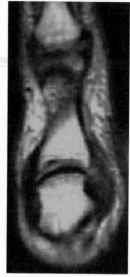

FIGURE 3.35A-1   **FIGURE 3.35B**

CLINICAL HISTORY

A 40-year-old man had persistent thumb pain following a skiing accident.

FINDINGS

Coronal T1- (Fig. 3.35A-1) and proton-density-weighted images (Fig. 3.35B) of the thumb show intermediate signal intensity within the ulnar collateral ligament of the first metacarpal phalangeal joint. The ligament is disrupted at its distal attachment at the base of the first proximal phalanx and is retracted proximally. The ligament remains deep to the adductor pollicis muscle aponeurosis (Fig. 3.35A-2, *arrow*).

DIAGNOSIS

Disruption of the ulnar collateral ligament (gamekeeper's thumb).

DISCUSSION

A "gamekeeper's thumb" refers to an acute or chronic injury of the ulnar collateral ligament. The term was originally used to describe an occupational injury in Scottish gamekeepers, who tore their ulnar collateral ligaments from chronic ligamentous strain while killing rabbits by twisting the neck of the animal (1–3). Nowadays, this hyperabduction injury is more commonly associated with skiing injury as the thumb catches in the strap of the ski pole during a fall. More than 50% of all skiing-related hand injuries are injuries of the ulnar collateral ligament (4). Other causes for a

gamekeeper's thumb are motor vehicle accidents, falls, break dancing, and other sports-related injuries.

The ulnar collateral ligament complex of the first metacarpophalangeal joint is composed of the ulnar collateral ligament proper and the accessory collateral ligaments. The collateral ligaments are continuous with the articular capsule and reinforce the capsule medially and laterally. The ulnar collateral ligament proper arises from the medial tubercle of the metacarpal condyle and passes volarly and obliquely to insert onto the base of the proximal phalanx near the attachment of the volar plate. The accessory ligament arises more volar to the proper ligament and inserts into the sides of the volar plate and the sesamoids. The ulnar collateral ligament is covered by the dorsal aponeurosis of the adductor pollicis muscle (2,3,5).

Injury of the ulnar collateral ligament is caused by a violent hyperabduction leading to a hyperextension injury of the first metacarpophalangeal joint. A fracture of the volar plate, usually through its thinner proximal part, is commonly seen as an associated injury. Tears of the ulnar collateral ligament most commonly occur near the distal insertion site but can occur proximally or in the mid substance of the ligament. If there is minimal retraction of the torn ligament, conservative management is currently the treatment of choice. When the ligament ruptures distally, the ligament can significantly retract proximally. In the presence of a retracted ligament, further abduction of the thumb may cause the torn ligament to displace superficial to the proximal margin of the adductor pollicis muscle aponeurosis. This finding is termed the *Stener lesion* and is observed in approximately 29% of the gamekeeper's thumb injuries (1). Interposition of the aponeurosis of the adductor pollicis muscle between the torn ligament and the phalangeal base prevents proper healing of the ligament, resulting in chronic functional instability. In the presence of a Stener lesion, surgical repair is indicated (2–5). Therefore proper distinction between a gamekeeper's thumb and a Stener lesion is important. The clinical diagnosis of a Stener lesion is difficult, especially in the presence of painful acute injury. Conventional radiographs can show if there is an avulsion fracture of the base of the first phalange or if the injury is limited to the soft tissues. Valgus stress radiographs are used to determine the degree of laxity and instability of the metacarpophalangeal joint. However, these examinations are not sufficiently accurate for the diagnosis of a Stener lesion.

MR imaging is excellent for the evaluation of a gamekeeper's thumb and can assess the position of the ligament relative to the adductor aponeurosis (4,5). The best plane of imaging is an oblique coronal plane, parallel to the course of the ligament. True orthogonal planes may fail to demonstrate the full course of the ligament on a single slice. On the oblique coronal images, the longitudinal direction of the entire ligament can be visualized in one or two images as a thin dark band spanning the medial side of the first metacarpophalangeal articulation. Disruption of the dark band indicates a rupture of the ligament. Interposition of the aponeurosis of the adductor pollicis muscle can also be identified in this plane. The presence of hemorrhage, effusion, and edema about the joint may be seen. In a chronic gamekeeper's thumb, the ligament appears thickened or attenuated and has irregular margins. Following a chronic injury, patients may complain of persistent pain, with or without clinical evidence of instability. In such cases, the tear in the ligament is often filled with intermediate-signal-enhancing granulation tissue that is preventing spontaneous healing.

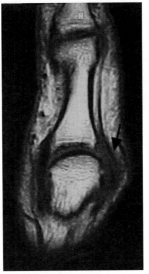

FIGURE 3.35A-2

REFERENCES

1. Hinke DH, Erickson SJ, Chamoy L, et al. Ulnar collateral ligament of the thumb: MR findings in cadavers, volunteers, and patients with ligamentous injury (gamekeeper's thumb). *AJR* 1994;163:1431–1434.
2. Ahn JM, Sartoris DJ, Kang HS, et al. Gamekeeper thumb: comparison of MR arthrography with conventional arthrography and MR imaging in cadavers. *Radiology* 1998;206:737–744.
3. O'Callaghan BI, Kohut G, Hoogewoud HM. Gamekeeper thumb: identification of the Stener lesion with US. *Radiology* 1994;192:477–480.
4. Hergan K, Mittler C, Oser W. Ulnar collateral ligament: differentiation of displaced and nondisplaced tears with US and MR imaging. *Radiology* 1995;194:65–71.
5. Masson JA, Golimbu CN, Grossman JA. MR imaging of the metacarpophalangeal joints. *Magn Reson Imaging Clin N Am* 1995;3:313–325.

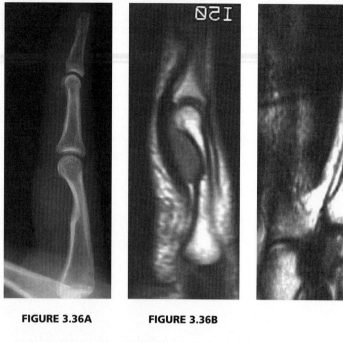

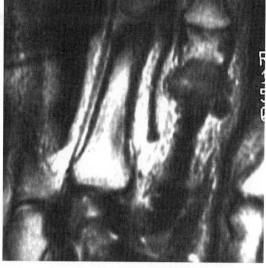

FIGURE 3.36A   **FIGURE 3.36B**   **FIGURE 3.36C**

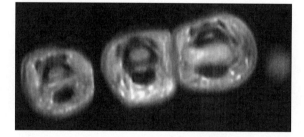

FIGURE 3.36D

CLINICAL HISTORY

A 62-year-old woman had a painless palpable mass on her third finger.

FINDINGS

The lateral radiograph of the third finger (Fig. 3.36A) shows a focal soft-tissue mass in the soft tissues volar to the proximal phalanx. The underlying bone has a smooth pressure erosion of the cortex, though the cortex remains intact (Fig. 3.36A). On the sagittal T1-weighted image (Fig. 3.36B), there is an ovoid homogeneous low-signal-intensity mass overlying the volar cortex of the proximal phalange, which is eroded. The underlying marrow space is attenuated but shows normal signal. The mass lies deep to the flexor digitorum longus tendon (Fig. 3.36B). The tendon is intact but is being bowed outward by the lesion. The mass has heterogeneous signal intensity with areas of low and high signal, though it remains predominantly low signal, even on the T2-weighted sequence (Fig. 3.36C). The lesion is intermediate signal intensity on the axial fat-suppressed proton-density-weighted image and is located between the proximal phalanx and the flexor tendon (Fig. 3.36D).

DIAGNOSIS

Giant cell tumor of the tendon sheath.

DISCUSSION

Giant cell tumor of the tendon sheath is also known as localized nodular synovitis or nonpigmented villonodular synovitis. It is the most common solid soft-tissue tumor of the hand and is the second most common tumor of the hand, second only to ganglion cysts in frequency (1–3). Other common sites of involvement by this lesion include the foot, ankle, knee, and hip. The lesion has a propensity to occur on the flexor surface of the second to fourth fingers, near the distal interphalangeal joint. It typically arises from the tendon sheath, though it can also be adherent to the tendon, palmar plate, capsular ligament, or joint. When the lesion is large, it can completely encircle the tendon or neurovascular bundles.

The histology of giant cell tumor is identical to that of pigmented villonodular synovitis, which occurs within the joint, so it is generally included in the general category of pigmented villonodular synovitis. These conditions are benign proliferations of round or polygonal histiocyte-like cells, associated with multinuclear giant foam- and hemosiderin-laden cells. Giant cell tumor of the tendon sheath occurs most commonly between the ages of 30 and 50 years. It is more common in women by a ratio of 3:2 to 2:1 (1,2). The lesion is slow growing and is usually painless. Occasionally, patients may experience mild numbness in the distal finger or notice a decreased range of motion. On physical examination, the lesions present as firm, lobulated, and nontender masses firmly fixed to the deep tissue. Treatment of giant cell tumor of the tendon sheath usually consists of local resection. Partial excision of the sheath or joint capsule is required to ensure complete removal of the tumor. Despite adequate excision of the lesion, recurrence rates can be as high as 30% (3).

Conventional radiographs are often normal; 50% of cases show a nonspecific soft-tissue mass. Approximately 8% to 14% of cases have pressure erosion of the adjacent bone or, less commonly, periosteal reaction of the adjacent bony cortex. Rarely, there may be calcification present within the lesion (1,3,4). On MR examination, giant cell tumor of the tendon sheath is typically a well-defined mass intimately associated with or encircling a tendon. On T1-weighted images, the lesion is homogeneous low signal intensity, similar to or less than that of muscle. On T2-weighted images, the lesion is predominantly low signal but may be heterogeneous. The signal characteristics are probably due to hemosiderin deposition or fibrotic tissues with hyperplastic stroma, large amount of collagen, and hyalinization of the lesions. Small areas of high signal intensity may be seen within the lesion on T2-weighted images and do not exclude the diagnosis of this lesion.

REFERENCES

1. Karasick D, Karasick S. Giant cell tumor of tendon sheath: spectrum of radiologic findings. *Skeletal Radiol* 1992;21:219–224.
2. Glowacki KA, Weiss AP. Giant cell tumors of tendon sheath. *Hand Clin* 1995;11:245–253.
3. Booth KC, Campbell GS, Chase DR. Giant cell tumor of tendon sheath with intraosseous invasion: a case report. *J Hand Surg [Am]* 1995;20:1000–1002.
4. Llauger J, Palmer J, Roson N, et al. Pigmented villonodular synovitis and giant cell tumors of the tendon sheath: radiologic and pathologic features. *AJR* 1999;172:1087–1091.

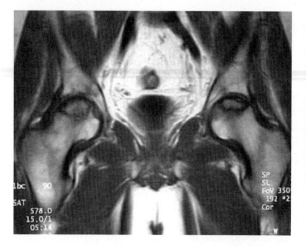

FIGURE 4.37A

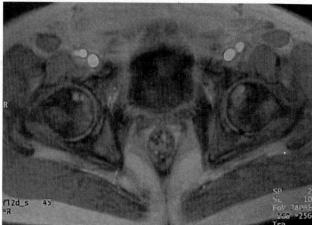

FIGURE 4.37B

CLINICAL HISTORY

A 49-year-old asthmatic male with a history of corticosteroid use complained of bilateral hip pain. The radiograph of the pelvis was normal.

FINDINGS

The T1-weighted coronal MR of the pelvis (Fig. 4.37A) shows linear bands of low signal in both femoral heads. These bands of low signal are in an arcuate configuration, isolating the subchondral regions of the femoral heads from the remaining marrow. The fatty signal marrow within the center of the low signal bands is presented. The axial T2*-weighted gradient-echo image (Fig. 4.37B) shows small, irregular foci of increased signal in the anterior portions of the femoral heads. The shape of the femoral heads remains normal.

DIAGNOSIS

Stage 2 avascular necrosis of both femoral heads.

DISCUSSION

The femoral head is the most frequent site of avascular necrosis (AVN) of bone. AVN is also commonly referred to as osteonecrosis, aseptic necrosis, or ischemic necrosis. There are numerous known etiologies for AVN, though up to one-third of cases are idiopathic. Posttraumatic AVN is caused by interruption of the blood supply to the femoral head by displaced intracapsular fractures of the femoral neck and following dislocation of the hip (1). Conditions associated with nontraumatic AVN include corticosteroid use, renal transplantation, irradiation, alcohol consumption, pancreatitis, sickle cell disease, Gaucher disease, dysbaric exposure, and other disorders interrupting the vascular supply to the bone marrow (1). In the United States, corticosteroid use is the most common cause of osteonecrosis of the femoral heads.

Avascular necrosis is staged according to the modified Ficat classification system, which divides AVN into five successive stages (2). Stage 0 (the silent hip) is incidentally detected AVN on MR or radionuclide imaging. This stage is both preclinical and preradiographic. In stage 1, there is development of clinical symptoms of progressive groin pain that radiates to the ipsilateral thigh, and limitation of motion of the hip joint. At this stage, conventional radiographs remain normal or only show nonspecific indistinctness of the trabeculae. In stage 2, symptoms persist or worsen and definite radiographic abnormalities are apparent in the femoral head, consisting of sclerosis, cystic changes, or mixed sclerosis and cystic changes. Stage 3 is characterized by the appearance of a crescentic subchondral fracture line, followed by subchondral collapse of the necrotic portion of the femoral head. Some classification systems subdivide stage 3 disease into two groups based on the presence or absence of collapse of the subchondral bone. The final stage in the Ficat classification, stage 4 disease, is the development of osteoarthritis of the hip joint caused by incongruity of the articular surface produced by collapse of the necrotic bone (2).

The choice of the various treatment options available for AVN varies, depending upon the severity of the patient's symptoms, the stage of the disease, and the extent of involvement of the weight-bearing portion of the head (3). The quantitative extent of the area of AVN can be calculated by measuring the percentage of the weight-bearing femoral subchondral cortex involved on the coronal MR images. The percentage of femoral head involvement is calculated by dividing the circumference of the involved femoral cortex abutting the acetabular roof by the entire acetabular weight-bearing area. When the subchondral bone of the femoral head is uninvolved, there is no involvement of the weight-bearing surface. In one study, collapse after core decompression developed in 43% of patients with 25% to 50% involvement, whereas 87% of patients with greater than 50% involvement of the femoral head developed collapse following the decompression procedure (3).

Therapy for early-stage osteonecrosis (stage 0 to 2) usually consists of limited weight bearing, core decompression, bone grafting, or femoral osteotomy to alter weight bearing (4,5). However, the long-term benefit of these treatments remains controversial. Newer surgical options for early-stage AVN include revascularization procedures using vascularized grafts obtained from the fibula or iliac bone (5). The treatment options for the later stages (stage 3 to 4) of femoral head osteonecrosis are limited to surgical replacement or arthrodesis of the joint (4). In stage 3 disease, femoral hemiarthroplasty can be performed, whereas patients with stage 4 disease, who have already developed osteoarthritis of the joint, typically require a total joint replacement.

REFERENCES

1. Meyers MH. Osteonecrosis of the femoral head: pathogenesis and long-term results of treatment. *Clin Orthop Rel Res* 1988;231:51–61.
2. Ficat RP. Idiopathic bone necrosis of the femoral head. *J Bone Joint Surg [Br]* 1985;67:3–9.
3. Beltran J, Knight CT, Zueler WA, et al. Core decompression for avascular necrosis of the femoral head: correlation between long-term results and preoperative MR staging. *Radiology* 1990;175:533–536.
4. Chang CC, Greenspan A, Gershwin ME. Osteonecrosis. Current perspectives on pathogenesis and treatment. *Semin Arthritis Rheum* 1993;23:47–69.
5. Wassenaar RP, Verburg H, Taconis WK, et al. Avascular osteonecrosis of the femoral head treated with a vascularized iliac bone graft: preliminary results and follow-up with radiography and MR imaging. *Radiographics* 1996;16:585–594.

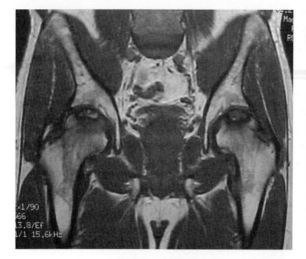

| FIGURE 4.38A | FIGURE 4.38B |

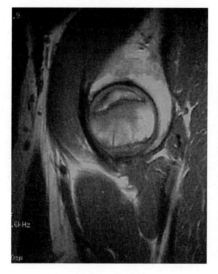

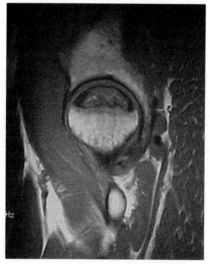

| FIGURE 4.38C | FIGURE 4.38D |

CLINICAL HISTORY

A 44-year-old alcoholic male complained of bilateral hip pain.

FINDINGS

The T1-weighted coronal image of the pelvis (Fig. 4.38A) shows curvilinear bands of low signal in the subchondral bone marrow. The central region of marrow within the low-signal lines remains of fat signal intensity. The corresponding fat-suppressed T2-weighted image (Fig. 4.38B) shows increased signal intensity within the femoral heads, with ex-tension of the abnormal signal into the femoral necks bilaterally. Sagittal T1-weighted images of the right hip (Fig. 4.38C) and left hip (Fig. 4.38D) also show the low-signal interface between the normal femoral marrow and the abnormal subchondral bone. The femoral heads retain their normal shape and are congruent with the acetabulum.

DIAGNOSIS

Bilateral avascular necrosis of the femoral heads.

DISCUSSION

MR imaging is the most sensitive and accurate modality for the diagnosis of avascular necrosis (AVN) of bone, particularly in the early stages of osteonecrosis (1,2). Changes within the bone marrow can be seen prior to the development of the radiographic finding of lysis, sclerosis, and subchondral collapse (3). MR imaging has become the screening modality of choice for the early diagnosis of this disorder. AVN of the femoral head is bilateral in up to 50% of cases. Therefore even when only one hip is symptomatic, MR imaging of both hips should be performed. The asymptomatic hip generally demonstrates an earlier stage of involvement when joint-preserving therapy is more successful (1).

The MR appearance of AVN of the femoral head correlates with the underlying pathologic changes taking place within the bone. Following the onset of vascular insufficiency, necrosis of different cell lines occurs sequentially, with initial necrosis of hematopoietic cells, followed by fat cells, and finally osteocytes (1,3). In very early AVN, the MR examination may be normal, presumably due to lack of any significant reactive edema, hemorrhage, or bone response (4). Dynamic contrast-enhanced MR shows lack of enhancement of the avascular marrow prior to the development of any abnormal MR findings on standard spin-echo and short tau inversion recovery (STIR) sequences (5). Dynamic contrast-enhanced MR is recommended for early diagnosis of osteonecrosis following an acute subcapital femoral neck fracture since conventional MR will not show changes for up to 1 week following devasculation of the marrow (5).

The earliest MR finding in AVN is nonspecific bone marrow edema, which can be extensive, even in the presence of a small infarct (6). Fortunately, this pattern of isolated edema without any focal associated MR features of osteonecrosis is quite rare. It may not be possible to distinguish this phase from idiopathic bone marrow edema unless one identifies a focal abnormality in the femoral head (3). Over a period of days, reactive changes at the margins of the infarct become apparent while the central region of infarction maintains normal fat signal. With high-resolution imaging, focal reactive changes can be recognized in the vast majority of patients with AVN, even if the predominant MR finding is bone marrow edema (3). This reactive zone is visualized as a line, band, or ring of low signal surrounding the area of infarcted bone (1,3). The reparative tissue at the interface, which is low signal intensity on both the T1-weighted and T2-weighted sequences, probably consists of peripheral fibrosis and/or thickened trabecular bone (3). Vascularized granulation tissue just inside the reactive bone results in a second band area of intermediate to high signal intensity on the T2-weighted images, producing the "double-line sign" of AVN (2). In the frequency encode direction, this appearance is often accentuated by a chemical shift misregistration artifact at the interface of the fat and the reparative tissue (2). This double-line sign is seen in up to 80% of patients with AVN of the femoral head, and it is a very specific indicator of osteonecrosis (2).

Subchondral fractures of the femoral head develop as the infarcted bone loses volume. These fractures weaken the subchondral bone and ultimately lead to collapse of the subchondral bone of the femoral head. The subchondral fracture is difficult to identify on the T1-weighted images. The fracture is most easily visible on T2-weighted images, where it appears as an arc of high signal intensity, probably representing edema or articular fluid within the cleft (3). The next stage of AVN is the development of collapse of the articular surface. Collapse develops initially in the anterosuperior portion of the head and results in loss of the normal spherical contour of the femoral head (3). The deformity of the femoral head and the resultant incongruity between the femoral head and acetabulum is best evaluated on high-resolution sagittal images (7). With longstanding collapse of the femoral head, the infarcted marrow often develops regions of fibrosis, producing low signal on the T2-weighted images (1). Superimposed changes of osteoarthritis are present at this final stage of the disease.

REFERENCES

1. Mitchell DG, Rao VM, Dalinka MK, et al. Femoral head avascular necrosis: correlation of MR imaging, radiographic staging, radionuclide imaging, and clinical findings. *Radiology* 1987;162:709–715.
2. Zurlo JV. The double-line sign. *Radiology* 1999;212:541–542.
3. Vande Berg B, Malghem J, Labaisse MA, et al. Avascular necrosis of the hip: comparison of contrast-enhanced and nonenhanced MR imaging with histologic correlation. *Radiology* 1992;182:445–450.
4. Speer KP, Spritzer CE, Harrelson JM, et al. Magnetic resonance imaging of the femoral head after acute intracapsular fracture of the femoral neck. *J Bone Joint Surg* 1990;72:98–103.
5. Nadel SN, Debatin JF, Richardson WJ, et al. Detection of acute avascular necrosis of the femoral head in dogs: dynamic contrast-enhanced MR imaging vs spin-echo and STIR sequences. *AJR* 1992;159:1255–1261.
6. Turner DA, Templeton AC, Selzer PM, et al. Femoral capital osteonecrosis: MR finding of diffuse marrow abnormalities without focal lesions. *Radiology* 1989;171:135–140.
7. Shuman WP, Castagno AA, Baron RL, et al. MR imaging of avascular necrosis of the femoral head: Value of small field-of-view sagittal surface-coil images. *AJR* 1988;150:1073–1078.

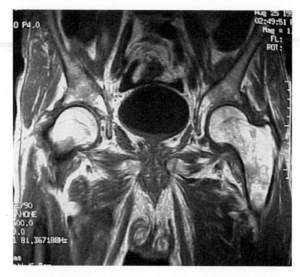

FIGURE 4.39A

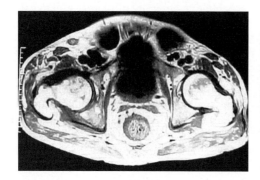

FIGURE 4.39B

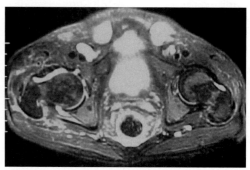

FIGURE 4.39C

CLINICAL HISTORY

A 74-year-old man with chronic liver failure and ascites complained of severe right hip pain and a high fever for the past 5 days.

FINDINGS

The T1-weighted coronal image of the pelvis shows no osseous abnormalities (Fig. 4.39A). On the axial T1-weighted image, there is an effusion within the right hip joint causing distention of the hip capsule (Fig. 4.39B). The fat-suppressed axial T2-weighted image (Fig. 4.39C) shows joint effusion as well as streaky high signal in the adjacent periarticular soft tissues. Incidental note is made of fluid in the inguinal canals bilaterally due to the patient's ascites.

DIAGNOSIS

Septic arthritis of the right hip with periarticular edema.

DISCUSSION

Septic arthritis can result from direct hematogenous spread of infection to the synovial membrane, spread from contiguous metaphyseal osteomyelitis, and direct inoculation of the joint. Septic arthritis secondary to adjacent osteomyelitis occurs most frequently in the infant hip (1). The metaphysis of the proximal femur lies within the joint capsule, and infection of the proximal femur can spread into the adjacent hip joint. In the lax joints of an infant, the accumulation of joint fluid can produce marked widening of the joint space and pathologic subluxation. In children and adults, hematogenous spread to the synovial articular lining is the most common mechanism responsible for septic arthritis.

Septic arthritis involves all age groups, though there is an increased frequency of this condition in the very young, the elderly, and the immunocompromised patient. Intravenous drug abusers and patients with underlying inflammatory arthropathies, such as rheumatoid arthritis, are at high risk for septic arthritis (1). *Staphylococcus aureus* is the most common organism responsible for articular infection in all age groups (1). In younger children, *Hemophilus influenzae* and group D streptococci are also common pathogens. Multifocal septic arthritis in young adults is suggestive of gonococcal arthritis. Septic arthritis secondary to tuberculosis and fungal diseases shows prominent osteoporosis, a slower rate of destruction, and less joint space narrowing than with pyogenic infection.

The most typical sites of hematogenous septic arthritis are the hip and knee articulations. The clinical symptoms consist of fever, local pain, and a limited range of motion of the involved joint. A tense joint effusion is generally present, associated with regional hyperemia resulting in swelling and redness of the overlying soft tissues. Diagnostic imaging plays a minor role in the initial diagnosis of septic arthritis, which is typically diagnosed on the basis of aspiration of the joint. Radiographic findings associated with septic arthritis include soft-tissue swelling and joint effusion, rapid osteoporosis, narrowing of the joint space due to erosion of cartilage, and marginal and central osseous erosions. In early septic arthritis, the joint may be widened by effusion, but it rapidly narrows as cartilage is eroded. Joint space loss is uniform and not accompanied by sclerosis or productive bone changes.

In the early stages of septic arthritis, MR imaging typically shows only a nonspecific joint effusion. In the hip joint, a large effusion can be associated with distention of the iliopsoas bursa, a rounded bursa that lies anterior to the hip joint in the femoral triangle and communicates with the joint in 10% to 15% of patients (2). Unlike bland sterile effusions, septic effusions often obliterate the intraarticular fat pads, such as the pulvinar in the acetabular fossa, and produce inflammation in the adjacent soft tissues (3). In chronic infection, synovial hypertrophy and debris within the joint may be apparent, leading to signal inhomogeneity on T2-weighted images. The inflamed synovium is irregular, inhomogeneous, and lower signal than bland joint fluid. Loculated pockets of fluid and enlarged periarticular bursa, sinus tracts, and soft-tissue abscesses can be seen in the adjacent soft tissues in neglected septic joint disease. Gadolinium enhancement results in enhancement of both the thickened synovium and the inflamed periarticular soft tissues.

The adjacent bones are usually normal in patients with septic arthritis. Mild or moderate amounts of reactive edema that can simulate osteomyelitis have been reported in up to 50% of patients with septic arthritis, even in the absence of histologic evidence of osseous infection (4). This reactive edema tends to be patchy, to be ill defined, and to involve both sides of the articulation symmetrically. MR distinction between reactive marrow edema and frank osteomyelitis can be difficult. Cortical integrity, the absence of erosions, and symmetric involvement on both sides of the joint suggest reactive edema. When septic arthritis is complicated by adjacent osteomyelitis, the changes predominate in one of the adjacent bones, and erosion of the subchondral bone and cortex are present (4).

REFERENCES

1. Resnick D. Infectious arthritis. *Semin Roentgenol* 1982;17:49–58.
2. Varma DGK, Richli WR, Charnsangavej C, et al. MR appearance of the distended iliopsoas bursa. *AJR* 1991;156:1025–1028.
3. Schweitzer ME, Falk A, Pathria MN, et al. MR imaging of the knee: Can changes in the intracapsular fat pads be used as a sign of synovial proliferation in the presence of an effusion? *AJR* 1993;160:823–826.
4. Erdman WA, Ramburro F, Jayson HT, et al. Osteomyelitis: characteristics and pitfalls of diagnosis with MR imaging. *Radiology* 1991;180:533–539.

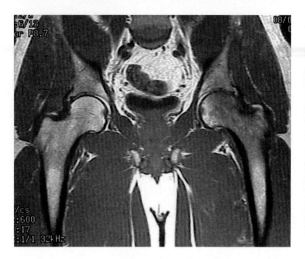

FIGURE 4.40A

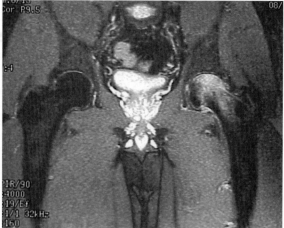

FIGURE 4.40B

CLINICAL HISTORY

A 42-year-old male complained of severe pain of his left hip that had been present for 3 weeks.

FINDINGS

The T1-weighted coronal MR (Fig. 4.40A) of the pelvis shows loss of the normal high signal of the bone marrow in the left femoral head and femoral neck to the level of the intertrochanteric ridge. The coronal fat-suppressed proton-density image (Fig. 4.40B) shows homogeneous high signal throughout the femoral head, neck, and intertrochanteric region, as well as a small joint effusion. No low-signal band is present within the femoral head.

DIAGNOSIS

Transient bone marrow edema of the left femoral head.

DISCUSSION

Transient idiopathic bone marrow of the femoral head is a common finding on MR imaging in adults with unexplained hip pain. The patient complains of the spontaneous abrupt onset of hip pain that is exacerbated by weight bearing. Three related syndromes, known as transient osteoporosis of the hip (TOH), regional migratory osteoporosis, and "transient bone marrow edema syndrome," all produce proximal femur bone marrow edema (1). All three have an identical MR appearance and self-limited clinical course.

Transient osteoporosis of the hip refers to the radiographic demonstration of focal osteoporosis of the proximal femur in addition to the presence of bone marrow edema. Despite the prominent demineralization of the bone, the joint space remains preserved. Regional migratory osteoporosis is a less common disorder in which multiple anatomic sites are affected sequentially (2). Resolution of marrow edema at the initial site is followed by the development of similar changes in other regions of the ipsilateral or contralateral extremity. The most recently described entity in this group of disorders has been designated as the *transient bone marrow edema syndrome* (1). This pattern has no radiographic findings and is diagnosed on the basis of clinical findings and abnormalities on MR imaging. This variant is presumably an earlier, milder, or previously unrecognized form of TOH (1).

The MR appearance of transient bone marrow edema is a homogeneous, well-marginated region of altered signal in the marrow of the femoral head, femoral neck, and intertrochanteric region (1,3). The edema shows diminished signal on T1-weighted images and increased signal on STIR- and T2-weighted images, particularly if fat-suppression techniques are employed. The edema may involve the entire femoral head or there may be sparing of some portions of the head, either anteriorly or posteriorly. The extent and distribution of the marrow edema can change on sequential MR studies (4). The cortex and osseous contour remain intact and the soft tissues are normal, though a small joint effusion is usually present during the acute period (3).

No low-signal band, ring, or double-line sign is seen in patients with idiopathic bone marrow edema, whereas such linear densities are typically present in patients with avascular necrosis of the femoral head. Rarely, acute avascular necrosis can present with diffuse signal abnormality in the femoral head and neck without characteristic linear defects, and can be difficult to distinguish from transient bone marrow edema (5). If symptoms persist or if the patient has risk factors for avascular necrosis, follow-up imaging in 6 to 12 weeks can be helpful to differentiate these two entities. By this time the changes in the bone marrow should be resolving in patients with transient bone marrow edema syndrome.

REFERENCES

1. Hayes CW, Conway WF, Daniel WW. MR imaging of bone marrow edema pattern: transient osteoporosis, transient bone marrow edema syndrome, or osteonecrosis. *Radiographics* 1993;13:1001–1011.
2. Schapira D. Transient osteoporosis of the hip. *Semin Arthritis Rheum* 1992;22:98–105.
3. Pathria MN, Deutsch AL, Wilcox D. MR of the pelvis and hip. In: Deutsch AL, Mink JH, eds., *MRI of the musculoskeletal system: a teaching file,* 2nd ed. New York: Lippincott-Raven, 1997:197–272.
4. Hauzeur J, Hanquinet S, Gevenois P, et al. Study of magnetic resonance imaging in transient osteoporosis of the hip. *J Rheumatol* 1991;18:1211–1217.
5. Turner DA, Templeton AC, Selzer PM, et al. Femoral capital osteonecrosis: MR finding of diffuse marrow abnormalities without focal lesions. *Radiology* 1989;17:135–140.

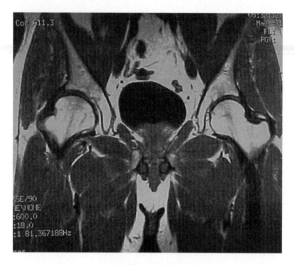

FIGURE 4.41A   **FIGURE 4.41B**

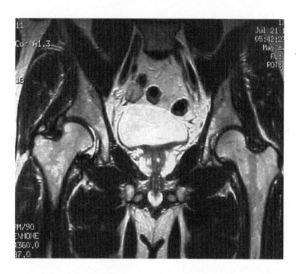

FIGURE 4.41C

CLINICAL HISTORY

A 42-year-old man with a remote history of Legg-Calve-Perthes disease complained of the recent onset of sharp right hip pain and a clicking sensation within the joint.

FINDINGS

The coronal T1-weighted image of the pelvis (Fig. 4.41A) shows deformity of the right femoral head due to remodeling of the femoral head and neck. The head is flattened and enlarged, and the femoral neck is short and broadened, consistent with the clinical history of childhood osteonecrosis. A more posterior coronal T1-weighted image

(Fig. 4.41B) shows thickening and increased signal within the superior labrum of the right hip joint. The corresponding coronal T2-weighted image (Fig. 4.41C) also shows the enlargement of the right hip labrum, which remains intermediate signal intensity with T2 weighting.

DIAGNOSIS

Tear of the acetabular labrum of the right hip associated with dysplasia of the hip due to remote Legg-Calve-Perthes disease.

DISCUSSION

Lesions of the acetabular labrum are a significant but underrecognized cause of hip pain in adults with dysplastic hip joints (1). The increased frequency of acetabular labral tears in patients with underlying acetabular dysplasia is thought to be due to uncovering of the lateral portion of the femoral head, resulting in excessive stress on the posterosuperior labrum (2). Less commonly, posttraumatic labral tears are observed and are typically caused by an acute injury in a high-performance athlete.

The patient with a torn acetabular labrum commonly complains of mechanical pain localized to the hip joint, variously described by the patient as sharp, catching, or associated with a clicking sensation. Less frequently, the pain resulting from an enlarged edematous labrum produces stretching of the capsule of the hip joint, mimicking sciatica as it radiates down the thigh (3). Labral tears can be managed conservatively by a period of no weight bearing or partial resection of the torn labrum (2). If untreated, labral tears may enlarge and result in premature secondary osteoarthrosis, and the formation of intraosseous and periacetabular ganglia. It is thought that the loss of congruity between the femoral head and acetabulum due to a labral tear leads to the development of premature osteoarthrosis (2).

Tears of the acetabular labrum produce no specific radiographic abnormality, though they can be recognized with conventional arthrography, MR imaging, and MR arthrography. Although arthroscopy and MR arthrography appear to be the most accurate methods for the diagnosis of tears of the acetabular labrum, there are findings on conventional MR imaging that afford noninvasive diagnosis (1,4). The normal labrum is a triangular structure of homogeneous low signal intensity located at the periphery of the acetabulum, thicker posterosuperiorly than in its anteroinferior portion (1,4). It is normally separated from the overlying capsule by a small recess, which is most prominent in the superior part of the joint. There is controversy regarding the existence of a normal sublabral sulcus between the labrum and the bone (4,5). Czerny et al. believe that there is no sublabral sulcus and that all linear regions of high signal in the substance of the labrum or at the labral-osseous junction should be considered a tear (4). Other authors believe that there is considerable variability in the size, shape, and signal of the normal labrum and that such a sulcus represents a normal variant (1,5). Further studies are necessary to clarify the normal appearance and variations of this structure.

Most tears of the labrum occur in the anterior, anterosuperior, or superior labrum. The anterosuperior labrum appears to be the site of tear in most patients with underlying hip dysplasia. However, in one small series comprised of younger patients with posttraumatic tears, the site of tear was predominantly in the posterosuperior portion (6). Linear tears of the labrum are typically longitudinal and difficult to identify on MR imaging in the absence of significant effusion or contrast material in the joint. Often tears of the labrum are associated with thickening and enlargement of the torn labrum, producing an intermediate-signal rounded mass in the region of the tear. The bulging edematous labrum often obliterates the normal recess between the hip capsule and the outer margin of the labrum. Ultimately, detachment of the torn labrum from the bone occurs, with separation of the thickened labrum from the osseous structures (4).

REFERENCES

1. Petersilge CA, Haque MA, Petersilge WJ, et al. Acetabular labral tears: evaluation with MR arthrography. *Radiology* 1996;200:231–235.
2. Dorrell JH, Catterall A. The torn acetabular labrum. *J Bone Joint Surg [Br]* 1986;68:400–403.
3. Ueo T, Hamabuchi M. Hip pain caused by cystic deformation of the labrum acetabulare. *Arthritis Rheum* 1984;27:947–950.
4. Czerny C, Hofmann S, Urban M, et al. MR arthrography of the adult acetabular capsular-labral complex: correlation with surgery and anatomy. *AJR* 1999;173:345–349.
5. Lecouvet FE, Vande Berg BC, Malghem J, et al. MR imaging of the acetabular labrum: variations in 200 asymptomatic hips. *AJR* 1996;167:1025–1028.
6. Ikeda T, Awaya G, Suzuki S, et al. Torn acetabular labrum in young patients: arthroscopic diagnosis and management. *J Bone Joint Surg* 1988;70:13–16.

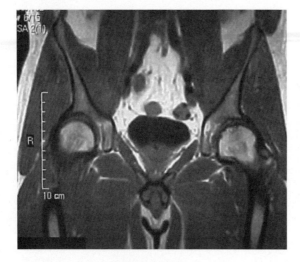
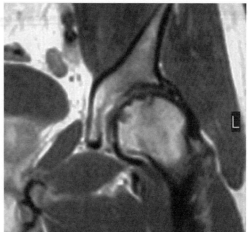

FIGURE 4.42A

FIGURE 4.42B

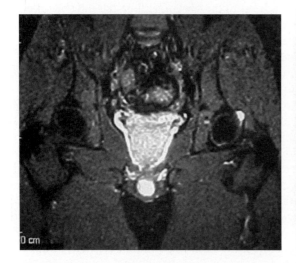
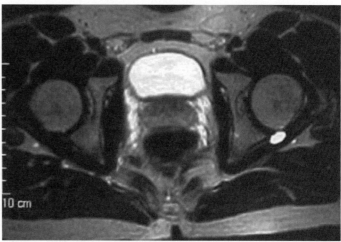

FIGURE 4.42C

FIGURE 4.42D

CLINICAL HISTORY

A 29-year-old male complained of left-sided hip pain. Radiographs of the pelvis showed mild bilateral hip dysplasia and early osteoarthritic changes of the left hip joint.

FINDINGS

The coronal T1-weighted image (Fig. 4.42A) shows mild bilateral hip dysplasia, with uncovering of the femoral heads bilaterally. A magnified image of the left hip from the coronal sequence shows detachment of the acetabular labrum from the underlying bone (Fig. 4.42B). The coronal STIR (Fig. 4.42C) and axial T2-weighted image (Fig. 4.42D) show a supraacetabular soft-tissue mass. The mass is well defined, homogeneous, and lobulated, and is located adjacent to the posterosuperior labrum. There is cortical irregularity and osteophyte formation along the surface of the left femoral head due to osteoarthritis.

DIAGNOSIS

Periacetabular ganglion adjacent to dysplastic hip with labral tear.

DISCUSSION

A ganglion is a common benign cystic lesion that differs from a synovial cyst by the absence of a true synovial cellular lining in ganglia and by the mucinous character of the internal contents of a ganglion cyst (1). The etiology of ganglia is unclear. It is believed that they develop following either synovial trauma or degenerative changes within the joint capsule, tendon sheath, or subchondral bone (2). Although most of the ganglia are adjacent to the synovium of either a joint capsule or a tendon sheath, nonarticular ganglion in intraosseous, subperiosteal, intramuscular, intratendinous, and subcutaneous locations have also been described (3,4). The hip region is a frequent site of development of intraosseous and soft-tissue ganglia, though it is much less commonly involved than the hand and wrist region (2,4). Most periacetabular ganglia are associated with tears of the acetabular labrum, a situation analogous with the cystic fluid collections seen along the scapula in patients with tears of the glenoid labrum.

Periacetabular ganglia are typically located superior to the hip joint, adjacent to the lateral cortex of the supraacetabular ilium. Conventional radiographs are usually normal, though mild hip dysplasia is frequently present in patients with nontraumatic labral tears. Uncommonly, the ganglion produces a well-defined extrinsic erosion of the lateral supraacetabular cortex. Rarely, small bubbles of intralesional nitrogen gas may be present within the lesion (3). Hip arthrography is insensitive for establishing the diagnosis as these ganglia usually do not become opacified by the injection of intraarticular contrast material, possibly due to a one-way valve effect. Computed tomography is also insensitive due to its limited soft-tissue contrast resolution, though large ganglia can be seen on the axial images above the acetabular roof.

Periacetabular ganglia are easily identified on MR imaging, particularly on T2-weighted images obtained in either the coronal or axial plane. Like ganglia in other locations, periacetabular ganglia are well marginated and have a spherical, elliptical, or lobulated shape (1,2). Thin-linear septae are frequently present within the substance of the lesion. On the T1-weighted images, ganglia are difficult to identify because their low-signal fluid content is difficult to distinguish from the hip capsule and overlying musculature. Ganglia are best seen on either fat-suppressed T2-weighted or STIR sequences due to their hyperintense signal on these sequences, allowing easy separation from the overlying musculature (2). With MR imaging, the contiguity of the ganglia with the acetabular joint capsule and labrum is also well shown. The underlying labrum can also be assessed.

REFERENCES

1. Abdelwahab IF, Kenan S, Hermann G, et al. Periosteal ganglia: CT and MR imaging features. *Radiology* 1993;188:245–248.
2. Haller J, Resnick D, Greenway G, et al. Juxtaacetabular ganglionic (or synovial) cysts: CT and MR features. *J Comput Assist Tomogr* 1989;13:976–983.
3. Silver DAT, Cassar-Pullicino VN, Morrissey BM, et al. Gas-containing ganglia of the hip. *Clin Radiol* 1992;46:257–260.
4. Feldman F, Singson RD, Staron RB. Magnetic resonance imaging of para-articular and ectopic ganglia. *Skeletal Radiol* 1989;18:353–358.

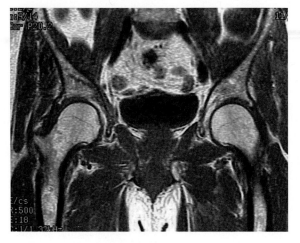

FIGURE 4.43A

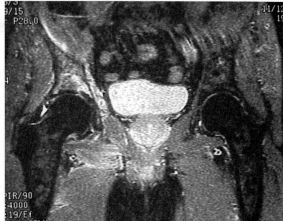

FIGURE 4.43B

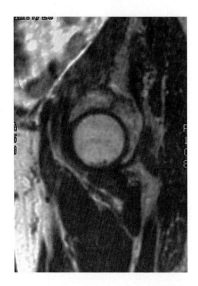

FIGURE 4.43C

CLINICAL HISTORY

A 69-year-old woman complained of gradually increasing pain in her right hip and groin.

FINDINGS

The coronal T1-weighted image of the pelvis shows multiple irregular low-signal intensities in the supraacetabular region of the right hip (Fig. 4.43A). The coronal STIR image shows high signal in the corresponding area, as well as abnormal increased signal in the obturator externus muscle (Fig. 4.43B). A sagittal T1-weighted image of the right hip again shows several low-signal lines above the acetabulum, with one vertical line extending into the roof of the acetabulum (Fig. 4.43C).

DIAGNOSIS

Insufficiency fracture of the acetabulum.

DISCUSSION

Insufficiency fractures develop in bone that is insufficient in its mineral or elastic resistance, most commonly in elderly females with senile osteoporosis and in patients who have undergone pelvic irradiation for visceral malignancy (1,2). Other risk factors for insufficiency fractures include osteomalacia, hyperparathyroidism, and rheumatoid arthritis (1). The typical clinical presentation is the onset of local pain without any antecedent trauma. In the acute phase, radiographs are normal. In the subacute and chronic phases, radiographs demonstrate reactive endosteal sclerosis at the fracture margins, but these osseous changes are easily overlooked due to overlying bowel gas and soft tissues. Bone scanning is more sensitive for early detection of pelvic insufficiency fractures and shows abnormal accumulation in the fracture site days or weeks prior to radiographic abnormalities (1). The scintigraphic finding of increased uptake is nonspecific and it is difficult to establish a definitive diagnosis of fracture.

MR imaging shows high sensitivity and allows visualization of the characteristic low-signal lines of a fracture. The MR appearance of insufficiency fracture depends on the stage on the bony injury. In the acute phase, fracture lines are poorly formed and the prominent finding is bone edema. As the fracture evolves and reactive sclerosis develops around the fracture, low-signal lines become visible, surrounded by wide areas of edema (3). Once the low-signal linear fracture line is identified, a confident diagnosis of insufficiency fracture can be made.

Supraacetabular insufficiency fractures are difficult to visualize on radiographs. These fractures, which are frequently bilateral, develop superior to the acetabulum and appear as an arched band of subchondral sclerosis oriented parallel to the acetabular roof (4). The curvilinear low-signal fracture line in the iliac bone is well seen on coronal and sagittal MR images, as is the surrounding marrow edema (5). The fracture line in the supraacetabular region may be difficult to see on axial imaging due to its predominantly horizontal orientation. Insufficiency fractures of the pelvis involve multiple sites in up to 50% to 85% of patients, so identification of an acetabular insufficiency fracture should prompt a thorough evaluation of the remainder of the pelvis. Other common locations for insufficiency fractures in the pelvis include the lateral alae of the sacrum, the pubic rami, and the parasymphyseal region (2–4).

REFERENCES

1. Daffner RH, Pavlov H. Stress fractures: current concepts. *AJR* 1992;159:245–252.
2. Blomlie V, Lien HH, Iversen T, et al. Radiation-induced insufficiency fractures of the sacrum: evaluation with MR imaging. *Radiology* 1993;188:241–244.
3. Brahme SK, Cervilla V, Vint V, et al. Magnetic resonance appearance of sacral insufficiency fractures. *Skeletal Radiol* 1990;19:489–493.
4. Cooper KL, Beabout JW, McLeod RA. Supraacetabular insufficiency fractures. *Radiology* 1985;157:15–17.
5. Grangier C, Garcia J, Howarth NR, et al. Role of MRI in the diagnosis of insufficiency fractures of the sacrum and acetabular roof. *Skeletal Radiol* 1997;26:517–524.

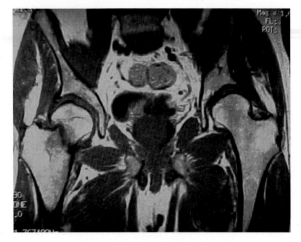

FIGURE 4.44A

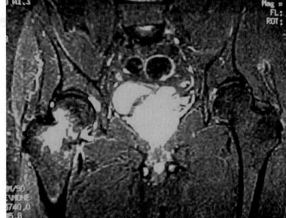

FIGURE 4.44B

CLINICAL HISTORY

This elderly man was unable to weight bear on the right leg following a fall. Radiographs obtained in the emergency room were interpreted as normal.

FINDINGS

The coronal T1-weighted image of the pelvis shows an irregular low-signal line traversing the right femoral neck (Fig. 4.44A). There is mild valgus angulation of the femoral neck at the site of the linear density. The fat-suppressed T2-weighted image shows high-signal edema in the right femoral neck (Fig. 4.44B). The linear band is less apparent on this sequence.

DIAGNOSIS

Radiographically occult fracture of the right femoral neck.

DISCUSSION

Relatively minor trauma can result in a fracture of the femoral neck in the elderly, osteoporotic patient. Conventional radiography can fail to demonstrate this important fracture when the underlying bone is severely demineralized, the femoral neck is poorly positioned or overpenetrated, and the fracture is minimally displaced. In 1989, Deutsch et al. described the use of MR imaging for the diagnosis of radiographically occult fractures of the proximal femur (1). Since that time, MR has become the imaging modality of choice for detection of a suspected hip fracture in the patient with posttraumatic pain, inability to weight bear, and normal radiographs. At many institutions, MR has replaced scintigraphy for the detection of a suspected hip fracture. MR has been shown to be as sensitive as scintigraphy for the diagnosis of occult osseous trauma of the femoral neck (2,3). Evans et al. compared MR imaging with scintigraphy (obtained more than 48 hours following injury) in 37 patients with traumatic hip pain and normal radiographs. MR was 100% accurate and showed eight femoral fractures, whereas only six were diagnosed on the bone scan (3). MR can be performed immediately following the injury, obviating the 48- to 72-hour delay considered necessary for scintigraphy (2). An additional advantage of MR imaging is its ability to provide an anatomic depiction of the fracture, such as its degree of angulation and displacement (2). Displacement and angulation are important features of the injury that impact its operative fixation. Fractures that show significant varus angulation or displacement have a high risk for avascular necrosis and are treated more aggressively than undisplaced fractures or those that show valgus impaction.

A routine MR pelvic examination will afford accurate depiction of the presence and anatomic configuration of a femoral fracture. A complete pelvic MR study can also assess the soft tissues for concomitant injury, such as muscle contusion or hematoma. However, the use of limited screening studies consisting of only one or two imaging sequences has also been emphasized for diagnosis of the simple presence or absence of a fracture of the femur. A low-cost screening MR examination, consisting of two sequences, is accurate and cost-effective for identifying the presence of significant osseous injury (4). At our institution, we obtain a fast STIR coronal sequence of the entire pelvis using the body coil. Subsequently, a small-field-of-view coronal T1-weighted sequence is obtained; the field of view is limited to the abnormal areas identified on the STIR sequence. The additional sagittal and axial imaging improves the depiction of the fracture anatomy but increases the cost of the examination.

The MR appearance of a traumatic fracture consists of an oblique or wavy linear band of low signal on T1-weighted spin-echo images, surrounded by low-signal edema. The normal physeal scar of the femoral head should not be mistaken for a fracture line. The physeal scar is curved, is very thin, has no edema surrounding it, and is located more proximally than the typical position of a subcapital fracture. On T2-weighted images, the fracture line remains low signal, whereas the surrounding edema becomes bright. On STIR, edema is the most prominent feature of the fracture (5). Hypointense fracture lines within the hyperintense marrow are seen in only 50% of patients. Routine MR imaging cannot detect the presence of diminished perfusion to the femoral head. At this time, MR cannot reliably predict the risk of avascular necrosis following a fracture of the femoral neck (6). Early detection of diminished perfusion requires IV contrast with dynamic assessment of marrow blood flow. Further work needs to be done on MR methods to evaluate bone marrow perfusion to that MR can help determine optimal therapy for the patient with a femoral neck fracture.

REFERENCES

1. Deutsch AL, Mink JH, Waxman AD. Occult fractures of the proximal femur: MR imaging. *Radiology* 1989;170:113–116.
2. Rizzo P, Gould ES, Lyden JP, et al. Diagnosis of occult fractures about the hip. *J Bone Joint Surg* 1993;75:395–401.
3. Evans PD, Wilson C, Lyons K. Comparison of MRI with bone scanning for suspected hip fracture in elderly patients. *J Bone Joint Surg [Br]* 1994;76:158–159.
4. Quinn SF, McCarthy JL. Prospective evaluation of patients with suspected hip fracture and indeterminate radiographs: use of T1-weighted MR images. *Radiology* 1993;187:469–471.
5. Berger PE, Ofstein RA, Jackson DW, et al. MRI demonstration of radiographically occult fractures. *Radiographics* 1989;9:407–436.
6. Speer KP, Spritzer CE, Harrelson JM, et al. Magnetic resonance imaging of the femoral head after acute intracapsular fracture of the femoral neck. *J Bone Joint Surg* 1990;72:98–103.

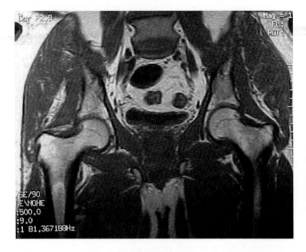

FIGURE 4.45A

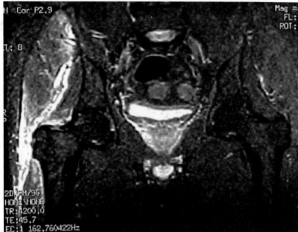

FIGURE 4.45B

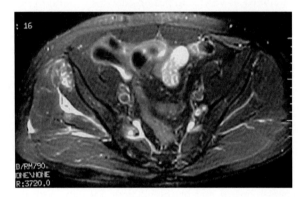

FIGURE 4.45C

CLINICAL HISTORY

A 55-year-old male described the spontaneous onset of severe pain overlying his right greater trochanter.

FINDINGS

The T1-weighted coronal image of the pelvis shows normal bone and no obvious abnormality (Fig. 4.45A). The T2-weighted coronal image (Fig. 4.45B) shows a large region of high signal in the soft tissues centered over the right greater trochanter. The region of high signal has no mass effect and appears ill defined, with feathery margins, consistent with edema. The gluteal tendons are obscured by the edema and difficult to define compared with the opposite side. An axial image obtained at the level of the buttock (Fig. 4.45C) shows high signal within the musculature of the gluteus medius and gluteus minimus muscles, as well as mild atrophy of the right gluteus medius muscle.

DIAGNOSIS

Trochanteric bursitis with underlying tendinopathy of the gluteal tendon.

DISCUSSION

The greater trochanteric pain syndrome is characterized by localized pain and point tenderness overlying the greater trochanter of the femur (1,2). The pain is typically unilateral and most common in middle-aged or elderly females. Causes of the greater trochanteric pain syndrome include inflammation of the synovium of the trochanteric bursa (trochanteric bursitis), tendinosis and tears of the gluteal muscle attachments on the trochanter, altered biomechanics, repetitive microtrauma, and crystal-induced inflammation (1,3). Clinically, cases of greater trochanteric pain syndrome are often referred to as *trochanteric bursitis,* though objective evidence of bursal inflammation is often lacking.

True trochanteric bursitis refers to inflammatory changes within the synovial lining of one or more of the bursal cavities overlying the greater trochanteric bursa. The largest of these bursae is the subgluteus maximus bursa, which lies inferior to the gluteus maximus muscle on the lateral aspect of the greater trochanter (2). Smaller bursa beneath the gluteus medius and the gluteus minimus tendons are located more cranially (2). Additional small bursae may also be present in this region. All the bursal cavities in this region are separate from the synovium of the hip joint.

The frequent association of trochanteric bursitis with underlying tendinosis or tears of the gluteus medius tendon has been emphasized (2,3). It has been suggested that tendinopathy or tears of the gluteal muscular attachments may be the direct cause of inflammation of the trochanteric bursa in a significant number of cases (2). The anatomy of the tendinous attachments of the gluteus medius and gluteus minimus muscles, and their relationship with the overlying trochanteric bursae, has been likened to that of the shoulder articulation. Therefore some authors use the term *rotator cuff lesions of the hip* to describe abnormalities in this area (3).

Diagnostic imaging plays a minor role in the management of patients with trochanteric bursitis. Imaging is typically reserved for recalcitrant cases that do not respond to the local injection of corticosteroids (2). The radiographic findings of trochanteric bursitis are limited to the occasional identification of calcification overlying the trochanteric and nonspecific bony proliferative changes in the region. Scintigraphy shows linear increased uptake along the outer surface of the trochanter, particularly on the blood pool images (4). MR imaging shows the changes of trochanteric bursitis, and affords assessment of the status of the underlying gluteal tendons (3,4). The STIR sequence appears to be most sensitive for identifying the increased signal produced by the soft-tissue inflammation (4). A distinct fluid collection can be seen due to distention of the bursae overlying the superolateral surface of the greater trochanter. The exact location of the fluid cavity depends on the specific bursa or bursae that are involved. Adjacent inflammatory changes in the soft tissues are commonly present. Tendinopathy and tears of the underlying gluteal tendons can also be identified on the MR images. The normal tendons of the gluteal muscles are best seen on the coronal and axial images. Thickening, increased signal, discontinuity, and absence of these tendons are all signs of underlying tendon pathology (2,3).

REFERENCES

1. Karpinski MRK, Piggott H. Greater trochanteric pain syndrome. *J Bone Joint Surg [Br]* 1985;67:762–763.
2. Kingzett-Taylor A, Tirman PFJ, Feller J, et al. Tendinosis and tears of gluteus medius and minimus muscles as a cause of hip pain: MR imaging findings. *AJR* 1999;173:1123–1126.
3. Chung CB, Robertson JE, Cho GJ, et al. Gluteus medius tendon tears and avulsive injuries in elderly women: imaging findings in six patients. *AJR* 1999;173:351–353.
4. Caruso FA, Toney MAO. Trochanteric bursitis: a case report of plain film, scintigraphic and MRI correlation. *Clin Nucl Med* 1994;19:393–395.

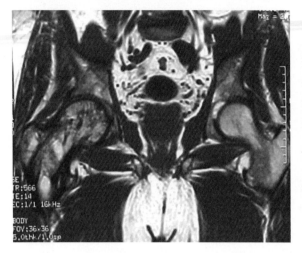

FIGURE 4.46A

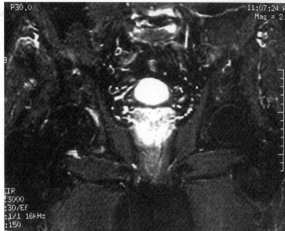

FIGURE 4.46B

CLINICAL HISTORY

A 71-year-old man had chronic pain of his right hip.

FINDINGS

The bone marrow is abnormal in the right femoral head, femoral neck, and proximal femoral shaft on the coronal T1-weighted image of the pelvis (Fig. 4.46A). The cortex is thickening and there are prominent low-signal trabeculae within the bone. Large amounts of marrow fat are interspersed within these irregular lines of low signal. There is a mild varus deformity of the proximal femur. The fat-suppressed T2-weighted image (Fig. 4.46B) shows normal marrow signal. The soft tissues are normal.

DIAGNOSIS

Paget disease of the right femur.

DISCUSSION

Paget disease is a common benign bone disorder of middle-aged and elderly adults, affecting 3% to 4% of individuals more than 40 years of age (1). Abnormal and excessive osseous remodeling is present, resulting in osseous enlargement, prominent disorganized trabeculae, and bone softening. The bone in Paget disease is weak and prone to fracture. Radiographs show osteosclerosis, cortical thickening, and prominent trabeculae. In the early phase of Paget disease, osteolysis may be the most prominent feature.

The most common sites of involvement are the ileum, sacrum, vertebrae, and calvarium (1). The proximal long bones, particularly the femur, are also frequently involved. Multifocal involvement is not uncommon, particularly in the very elderly patient with long-standing Paget disease. Paget disease is frequently asymptomatic or associated with mild local pain. The most serious complication of Paget disease is the development of Paget sarcoma, a virulent neoplasm with a high mortality rate (1,2).

Because of its high prevalence, Paget disease is commonly present on MR imaging of the pelvis. The diagnosis is often not considered when marrow disease of the pelvis or femur is identified on MR imaging (3). The osseous changes of Paget disease are less obvious on MR than they appear on radiographs or computed tomography. Cortical thickening and trabecular prominence appear low signal on all imaging sequences. The cortical thickening can be profound and produce an undulating contour of the endosteal cortex (4).

The appearance of the medullary cavity is variable in Paget disease. Normal-appearing fatty marrow, focal areas of fatty change, or soft-tissue material resembling neoplastic tissue can all be seen, depending on the phase of the disease (4). In active disease, multiple punctate intramedullary lesions that are low signal on T1-weighted images and increase in signal on T2-weighted images can be seen. These nodular areas represent areas of fibrovascular tissue that resembles granulation tissue (4). As the disease becomes quiescent, the trabecular coarsening is more prominent and the marrow returns to a more normal appearance. Cystlike areas of fat are surrounded by thickened cortical bone and interspersed with thickened, irregular trabeculae. The finding of persistent fat signal in an area of osseous sclerosis and trabecular thickening is highly suggestive of Paget disease (3,5).

REFERENCES

1. Resnick D. Paget disease of bone: current status and a look back to 1943 and earlier. *AJR* 1988;150:249–256.
2. Moore TE, King AR, Kathol MH, et al. Sarcoma in Paget disease of bone: clinical, radiologic, and pathologic features in 22 cases. *AJR* 1991;156:1199–1203.
3. Pathria MN, Deutsch AL, Wilcox D. MR of the pelvis and hip. In: Deutsch AL, Mink JH, eds., *MRI of the musculoskeletal system: a teaching file,* 2nd ed. New York: Lippincott-Raven, 1997:197–272.
4. Roberts MC, Kressel HY, Fallon MD, et al. Paget disease: MR imaging findings. *Radiology* 1989;173:341–345.
5. Kaufman GA, Sundaram M, McDonald DJ. Magnetic resonance imaging in symptomatic Paget's disease. *Skeletal Radiol* 1991;20:413–418.

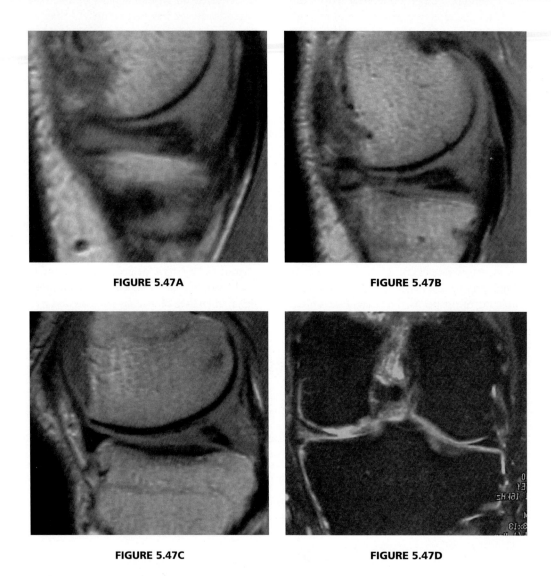

FIGURE 5.47A

FIGURE 5.47B

FIGURE 5.47C

FIGURE 5.47D

CLINICAL HISTORY

A 40-year-old male complained of persistent medial knee pain following a skiing injury.

FINDINGS

Sagittal proton-density-weighted images of the knee show linear increased signal intensity within the posterior horn and anterior horn of the medial meniscus (Fig. 5.47A–C). This increased signal extends all the way to the inferior free edge of the meniscal substance. The anterior horn of the medial meniscus shows normal morphology and low signal intensity (Fig. 5.47C). A linear region of increased signal is also seen on the coronal fat-suppressed proton-density image (Fig. 5.47D).

DIAGNOSIS

Tear of the posterior horn of the medial meniscus.

DISCUSSION

Magnetic resonance imaging has been shown to be highly accurate for the diagnosis of meniscal pathology. The medial and lateral menisci of the knee are fibrocartilaginous disks located between their respective femoral condyles and tibial plateaus. They act as cushions between these osseous structures and facilitate motion of the joint. The menisci cover the anterior, peripheral, and posterior articular surfaces of the tibial plateaus. Normally, there is no meniscal tissue covering their central aspects.

The lateral femoral meniscus is circular and crescentic. The width of the lateral meniscus is quite constant from anterior to posterior. The thickest portion is at the periphery of the meniscus, and it tapers to a millimeter at its inner margin (1,2). The lateral meniscus is attached to the capsule anteriorly and in its midportion, but there is no attachment posteriorly where the popliteus tendon traverses the joint. The medial meniscus is semicircular and crescentic in shape. Its anteroposterior dimension is almost twice that of the lateral meniscus. The medial meniscus is not uniform in size and has a posterior horn that is larger than its midportion and anterior horn (2). Unlike the lateral meniscus, which is loosely attached to the joint capsule, the medial meniscus is firmly attached to the capsule around its entire periphery and is therefore less mobile.

Meniscal tears may be degenerative or traumatic. Traumatic tears tend to be vertical and occur in younger people. Degenerative tears tend to be horizontal and occur in older people. However, there is considerable overlap in the morphology of these two types of tears, and it is not possible to distinguish them reliably based solely on the MR imaging findings (2).

Different classification systems have been used to describe the menisci on MR imaging. The most popular classification describes the menisci using a three-grade system (3). The normal meniscus is low signal throughout its substance on all MR imaging sequences. The grade 1 meniscus contains small irregular rounded regions of intermediate or high signal intensity that do not extend to the surface of the meniscus. The grade 2 meniscus shows linear signal alterations that are contained within the meniscus and do not extend to the meniscal surface. Grade 1 or grade 2 intrameniscal signal is considered to be due to either a normal variation or age-related degeneration of the meniscus (4–6), but it does not represent a meniscal tear (7). The grade 3 meniscus contains regions of abnormal increased signal intensity that extend all the way to the free edge of the meniscus. This appearance is strongly associated with a tear of the meniscus (8). This case is an example of a grade 3 meniscus where the increased signal intensity extends to the inferior free edge of the posterior horn of the medial meniscus.

REFERENCES

1. Firooznia H, Golimbu C, Rafii M. MR imaging of the menisci. *Magn Reson Imaging Clin North Am* 1994;2:325–347.
2. Resnick D. Knee. In: Resnick D, Kang HS, eds. *Internal derangements of joints.* Philadelphia: WB Saunders, 1997:595–633.
3. Crues JV, Mink J, Levy LT, et al. Meniscal tears of the knee: accuracy of MR imaging. *Radiology* 1987;164:445-448.
4. Quinn SE. Meniscal tear: pathological correlation with MR imaging. *Radiology* 1988;166:580–581.
5. Stoller DW, Martin C, Crues JV, et al. Meiscal tears: pathologic correlation with MR imaging. *Radiology* 1987;163:731–735.
6. Hajek PC, Gylys-Morin VM, Baker LL, et al. The high signal intensity meniscus of the knee: magnetic resonance evaluation and *in vivo* correlation. *Invest Radiol* 1987;22:883–890.
7. Kaplan PA, Nelson NL, Garvin KL, et al. MR of the knee: the significance of high signal in the meniscus that does not clearly extend to the surface. *AJR* 1991;156:333–336.
8. De Smet AA, Norris MA, Yandow DR, et al. MR diagnosis of meniscal tears of the knee: importance of high signal in the meniscus that extends to the surface. *AJR* 1993;161:101–107.

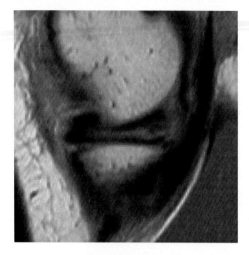

FIGURE 5.48A

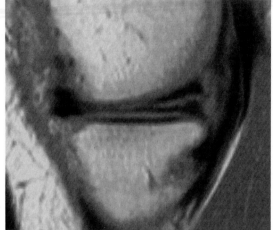

FIGURE 5.48B

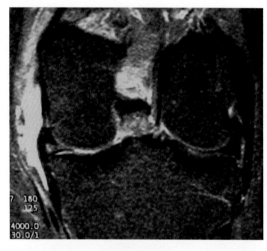

FIGURE 5.48C

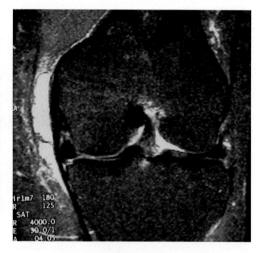

FIGURE 5.48D

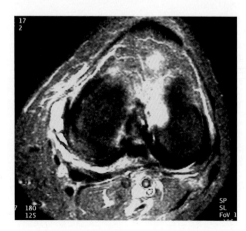

FIGURE 5.48E

CLINICAL HISTORY

Pain and swelling at the medial joint line of the knee.

FINDINGS

The sagittal proton-density-weighted images (Fig. 5.48A–B) of the posterior horn and middle portion of the medial meniscus show linear high signal that extends to its inferior free edge, indicating a meniscal tear. The fat-suppressed coronal proton-density image (Fig. 5.48C) also demonstrates an irregular medial meniscus with linear high signal within its substance. Adjacent to the torn meniscus, there is a lobulated fluid-filled mass that extends anteriorly to lie superficial to the medial collateral ligament (Fig. 5.48D–E).

DIAGNOSIS

Horizontal tear of the medial meniscus with an associated meniscal cyst.

DISCUSSION

Meniscal cysts are benign homogeneous fluid-filled collections that are typically seen in association with a meniscal tear (1). They are a complication of those meniscal tears that extend to the joint capsule (2), thereby allowing articular synovial fluid to extend through the tear and accumulate in the capsular and pericapsular tissues. In some patients, this repetitive accumulation of fluid leads to the development of an encapsulated cyst (3). Meniscal cysts may be asymptomatic, result in local pain, or present as a palpable mass. The cyst is typically tense and is often mistaken for a solid mass on palpation. Long-standing meniscal cysts can even result in pressure erosion of the adjacent tibial cortex (2).

Most meniscal cysts are located at the joint line, immediately adjacent to a meniscal tear. They occur with equal frequency on the medial and lateral sides of the knee, though lateral meniscal cysts are more likely to become symptomatic (4). Lateral meniscal cysts tend to be smaller than medial meniscal cysts and lie immediately overlying the meniscus, either anterior or posterior to the fibular collateral ligament. Medial meniscal cysts can be quite large but they are often asymptomatic. Medial cysts can dissect through the joint capsule and the pericapsular tissues to lie some distance away from the meniscus (4). They typically exit the capsule posteriorly and extend anteriorly to lie superficial to the medial collateral ligament. Less commonly, meniscal cysts can extend into Hoffa's (retropatellar) fat pad (Fig. 5.48F–G).

Meniscal cysts typically resolve spontaneously following resection or repair of the underlying meniscal tear. Underlying meniscal pathology needs to be corrected in order to prevent recurrence of the cyst (1). Cyst removal, cyst aspiration, and injection of steroids have all been employed to treat symptomatic cysts, but they tend to recur unless the underlying meniscal pathology is corrected.

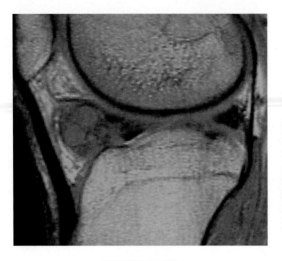

FIGURE 5.48F

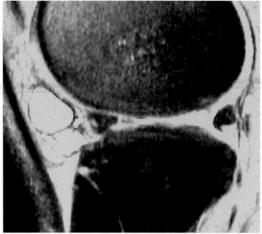

FIGURE 5.48G

REFERENCES

1. Lantz B, Singer KM. Meniscal cysts. *Clin Sports Med* 1990;9:707–725.
2. Juhng SK, Lenchik L, Won JJ. Tibial plateau erosions associated with lateral meniscal cysts. *Skeletal Radiol* 1998;27:288–290.
3. Tyson LL, Daughters TC Jr, Ryu RK, et al. MRI appearance of meniscal cysts. *Skeletal Radiol* 1995;24:421–424.
4. Resnick D. Knee. In: Resnick D, Kang HS, eds. *Internal derangements of joints.* Philadelphia: WB Saunders, 1997:624–625.

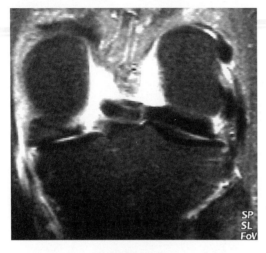

FIGURE 5.49A

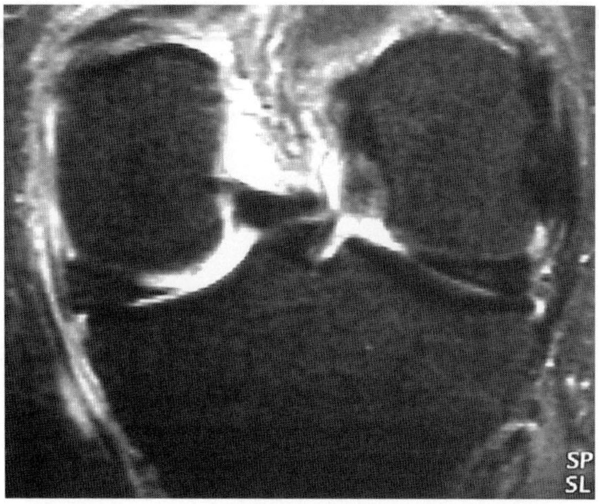

FIGURE 5.49B

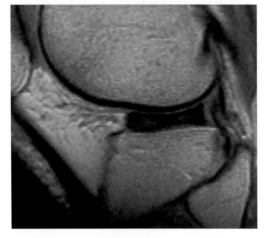

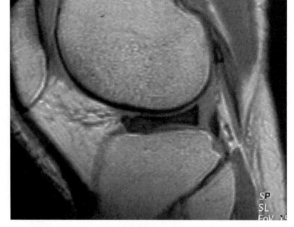

FIGURE 5.49C

FIGURE 5.49D

CLINICAL HISTORY

Medial and lateral knee pain. Evaluate for internal derangement.

FINDINGS

Sagittal and coronal images (Fig. 5.49A–B) show enlargement of the lateral meniscus, which is thicker than normal and extends medially toward the intercondylar notch. On the sagittal images, a bow-tie appearance of the lateral meniscus was present on five consecutive images. Abnormal linear signal intensity is present in the lateral meniscus (Fig. 5.49C–D). The increased signal extends to the inferior surface in the lateral meniscus, indicating a meniscal tear.

DIAGNOSIS

Discoid lateral menisci, with tear of the lateral meniscus.

DISCUSSION

A discoid meniscus is a dysplastic meniscus that has a broad disklike configuration rather than a normal semilunar shape. Although many different shapes of dysplastic menisci have been described (1), there is no uniform classification system for the discoid meniscus. The morphologies are typically classified into complete and incomplete forms based on the size of the meniscus, and the Wrisberg ligament type in which the posterior capsular attachment is lacking, resulting in a hypermobile meniscus (2–6). Complete and incomplete discoid menisci usually do not require surgical intervention unless a tear is present. The Wrisberg ligament type requires repair with saucerization of the meniscus (5).

On MR imaging, the discoid meniscus is best seen on coronal and sagittal images. On sagittal images, the normal meniscus usually has a bow-tie appearance on only two consecutive images at the peripheral aspect of the knee. The presence of a bow tie on three or more contiguous images is suggestive of discoid morphology. The height of the meniscus is also often greater than normal (7); this appearance can be associated with cupping and depression of the adjacent tibial plateau. On the coronal images, the discoid meniscus has a transverse width of 14 mm or greater (8), with the fibrocartilage extending toward intercondylar notch.

The criteria for MR diagnosis of a discoid meniscal tear are somewhat different than for a conventional meniscus. In a discoid meniscus, increased intrameniscal signal that does not extend all the way to the free edge of the meniscus frequently represents a symptomatic intrasubstance tear (9,10). Unlike a conventional meniscus, signal does not have to extend to the free edge of the meniscus in order to diagnose a meniscal tear.

REFERENCES

1. Weiner B, Rosenberg N. Discoid medial meniscus associations with bone changes in the tibia. *J Bone Joint Surg Am* 1974;56:171.
2. Monllau JC, Leon A, Cugat R, et al. Ring-shaped lateral meniscus. *Arthroscopy* 1998;14:502–504.
3. Stilli S, Di Gennaro GL, Marchiodi L, et al. Arthroscopic surgery of the discoid meniscus during childhood. *Chir Organi Mov* 1997;82:335–340.
4. Pellacci F, Montanari G, Prosperi P, et al. Lateral discoid meniscus: treatment and results. *Arthroscopy* 1992;8:526–530.
5. Woods GW, Whelan JM. Discoid meniscus. *Clin Sports Med* 1990;9:695–706.
6. Ikeuchi H. Meniscus surgery using the Watanabe arthroscope. *Orthop Clin North Am* 1979;10:629–642.
7. Silverman JM, Mink JH, Deutsch AL. Discoid menisci of the knee: MR imaging appearance. *Radiology* 1989;173:351–354.
8. Araki Y, Yamamoto H, Nakamura H, et al. MR diagnosis of discoid lateral menisci of the knee. *Eur J Radiol* 1994;18:92–95.
9. Hamada M, Shino K, Kawano K, et al. Usefulness of magnetic resonance imaging for detecting intrasubstance tear and/or degeneration of lateral discoid meniscus. *Arthroscopy* 1994;10:645–653.
10. Connolly B, Babyn PS, Wright JG, et al. Discoid meniscus in children: magnetic resonance imaging characteristics. *Can Assoc Radiol J* 1996;47:347–354.

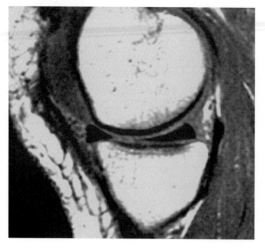

FIGURE 5.50A

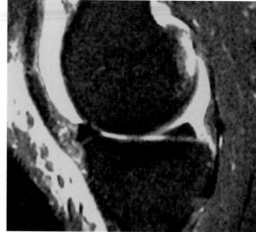

FIGURE 5.50B-1

CLINICAL HISTORY

Medial knee pain following injury.

FINDINGS

The sagittal proton-density-weighted image (Fig. 5.50A) and the corresponding fat-suppressed T2-weighted image show normal morphology of the medial meniscus. There is an abnormal band of fluid (Fig. 5.50A–B-1) completely separating the posterior horn of the medial meniscus from the joint capsule (Fig. 5.50B-2, *arrow*). A large joint effusion and anterior soft-tissue edema are also present.

DIAGNOSIS

Medial meniscocapsular separation.

DISCUSSION

Meniscocapsular separation refers to detachment of the meniscus from the adjacent joint capsule. The most common location for this injury is the capsular attachment of the posterior horn of the medial meniscus. The attachment of the posterior medial meniscus to the capsule and tibia is formed by the meniscotibial ligament, part of the medial capsular ligament. This ligament is vulnerable to tearing, leading to detachment of the meniscus from the capsule (1).

On MR imaging, meniscocapsular separation is best seen on T2-weighted sagittal and coronal images. MR finding of meniscocapsular separation includes the presence of fluid interposed between the meniscus and joint, displacement of the posterior horn of the medial meniscus by 5 mm or more from the capsule, and uncovering of the posterior tibial car-

tilage. Only the first of these signs—namely, fluid completely separating the meniscus from the capsule—has high specificity for this injury. The lateral meniscus has a normal dehiscence posteriorly for the popliteus tendon, so continuous fluid in this location is a normal finding.

The accuracy of MR for meniscocapsular separation is relatively low compared with its accuracy for meniscal tears (3). A peripheral tear of the meniscus can be difficult to distinguish from meniscocapsular separation, though some orthopedic surgeons consider these to be related injuries. The presence of prominent normal meniscocapsular recesses, a large joint effusion, and tibial collateral ligament bursitis can simulate meniscocapsular separation on MR imaging (4).

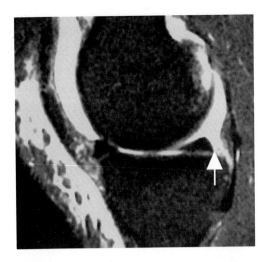

FIGURE 5.50B-2

REFERENCES

1. Stoller DW, Cannon WD Jr, Anderson LJ. The knee. In: Stoller DW, ed. *Magnetic resonance imaging in orthopedics and sports medicine,* 2nd ed. Philadelphia: Lippincott-Raven, 1996:Chapter 7.
2. De Maeseneer M, Lenchik L, Starok M, et al. Normal and abnormal medial meniscocapsular structures: MR imaging and sonography in cadavers. *AJR* 1998;171:969–976.
3. Rubin DA, Britton CA, Towers JD, et al. Are MR imaging signs of meniscocapsular separation valid? *Radiology* 1996;201:829–836.
4. Lee JK, Yao L. Tibial collateral ligament bursa: MR imaging. *Radiology* 1991;178:855–857.

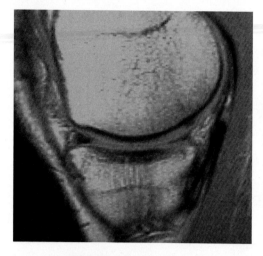

FIGURE 5.51A

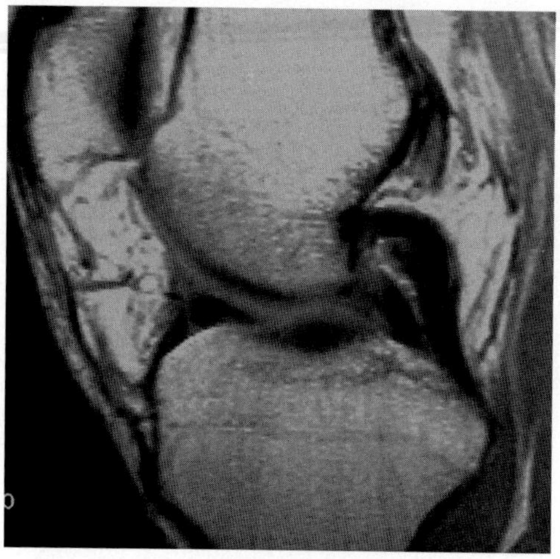

FIGURE 5.51B-1

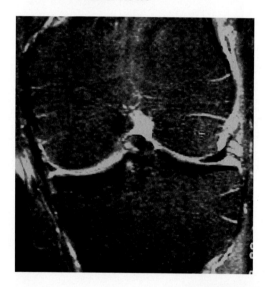

FIGURE 5.51C-1

CLINICAL HISTORY

Persistent medial knee pain with clicking and locking sensation after acute knee injury.

FINDINGS

A sagittal proton-density-weighted image of the medial knee joint (Fig. 5.51A) illustrates irregularity and severe truncation of the posterior horn of the medial meniscus. The normal bow-tie configuration of the meniscus is absent and the anterior horn is blunted and irregular. On the more central sagittal image, a low-signal-intensity band (Fig. 5.51B-2, *arrow*) is seen just inferior to the posterior cruciate ligament (PCL). On the coronal fat-suppressed proton-density image, a small fragment of low signal intensity is displaced into the region of the intercondylar notch just beneath the posterior cruciate ligament (Fig. 5.51C-2, *arrow*).

DIAGNOSIS

Bucket-handle tear of the medial meniscus.

DISCUSSION

A bucket-handle tear of the meniscus is a vertical or oblique tear that extends longitudinally along the long axis of the meniscus. The inner fragment is displaced away from the residual peripheral meniscus toward the intercondylar notch (1). This type of tear is more common in young adults and is more common in the medial meniscus (2). The sensitivity for diagnosis of bucket-handle tears on MR examination is relatively low because the peripheral nondisplaced component may appear relatively normal, showing only subtle truncation or irregularity of its inner margin (1). It is important to recognize the diminished size of the residual meniscus and identify the centrally displaced fragment in order to diagnose this type of tear accurately. When the inner fragment is displaced centrally, it typically lies inferior and anterior to the posterior cruciate ligament, giving the appearance of two posterior cruciate ligaments ("double PCL sign") (3). Other findings of a bucket-handle meniscal tear on MR include the "bow-tie sign" (4), where the normal bow-tie configuration of the peripheral meniscus on sagittal images is absent or seen on only one image due to central displacement of the meniscal material and the "flipped meniscus sign," which is more common with tears of the lateral meniscus (5).

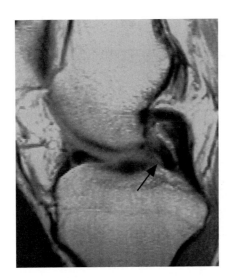

FIGURE 5.51B-2

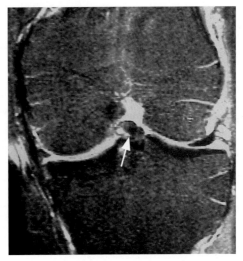

FIGURE 5.51C-2

REFERENCES

1. Singson RD, Feldman F, Staron R, et al. MR imaging of displaced bucket-handle tear of the medial meniscus [see comments]. *AJR* 1991;156:121–124.
2. Resnick D. Knee. In: Resnick D, Kang HS, eds. *Internal derangements of joints.* Philadelphia: WB Saunders, 1997:620–623.
3. Weiss KL, Morehouse HT, Levy IM. Sagittal MR images of the knee: a low-signal band parallel to the posterior cruciate ligament caused by a displaced bucket-handle tear. *AJR* 1991;156:117–119.
4. Helms CA, Laorr A, Cannon WD, Jr. The absent bow tie sign in bucket-handle tears of the menisci in the knee. *AJR* 1998;170:57–61.
5. Wright DH, De Smet AA, Norris M. Bucket-handle tears of the medial and lateral menisci of the knee: value of MR imaging in detecting displaced fragments. *AJR* 1995;165:621–625.

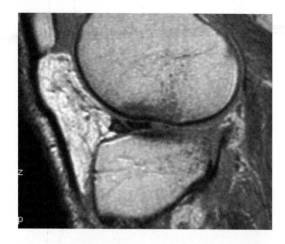

FIGURE 5.52A

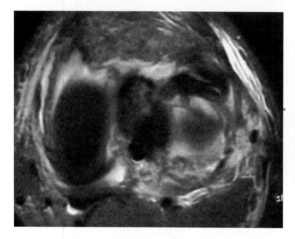

FIGURE 5.52B-1

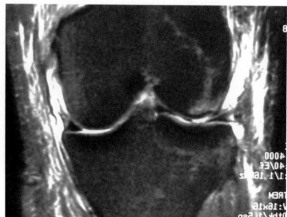

FIGURE 5.52C-1

CLINICAL HISTORY

Injured knee while playing sports.

FINDINGS

The proton-density-weighted sagittal image through the lateral joint space shows absence of the posterior horn of the lateral meniscus. Anteriorly, there are two triangular low-signal meniscal structures (Fig. 5.52A). The axial fat-suppressed proton-density image shows the posterior horn of the lateral meniscus displaced and folded over into the anterior aspect of the joint, lying anterior to the anterior horn of the meniscus (Fig. 5.52B-2, *arrow*). On the coronal fat-suppressed T2-weighted image, a torn disk fragment is seen in the inner aspect of the joint, just superior to the tibial spine (Fig. 5.52C-2, *arrow*). Abnormal high signal is present within the torn medial collateral ligament and lateral collateral ligament, as well as in the adjacent soft tissues (Fig. 5.52C-2). In addition, an anterior cruciate ligament (ACL) tear and bone marrow edema of the lateral femoral condyle and tibial plateau were present (not illustrated).

DIAGNOSIS

Bucket-handle tear of the lateral meniscus, associated with extensive ligament injury.

DISCUSSION

Displacement of a torn meniscal fragment into the anterior or posterior results in the "flipped meniscus sign" illustrated in this case. Unlike the "double posterior cruciate ligament sign," which is seen in association with bucket-handle tears of the medial meniscus, the flipped meniscus sign can be present in bucket-handle tears of either the medial or lateral meniscus (1,2). This appearance is due to displacement of a torn posterior meniscal fragment into the anterior aspect of the knee. The displaced fragment may be located on top of or lie in front of the anterior horn of the meniscus (3). On sagittal images, the anterior horn appears abnormally larger (8 mm or greater) (2) or appears elongated, with a small separation between two fragments (3). The posterior horn appears too small or is absent.

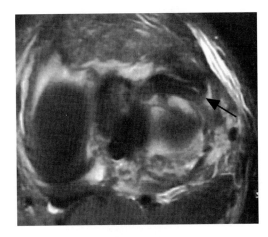

FIGURE 5.52B-2

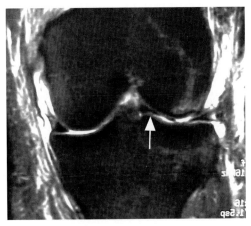

FIGURE 5.52C-2

REFERENCES

1. Wright DH, De Smet AA, Norris M. Bucket-handle tears of the medial and lateral menisci of the knee: value of MR imaging in detecting displaced fragments. *AJR* 1995;165:621–625.
2. Haramati N, Staron RB, Rubin S, et al. The flipped meniscus sign. *Skeletal Radiol* 1993;22:273–277.
3. Resnick D. Knee. In: Resnick D, Kang HS, eds. *Internal derangements of joints.* Philadelphia: WB Saunders, 1997:620–623.

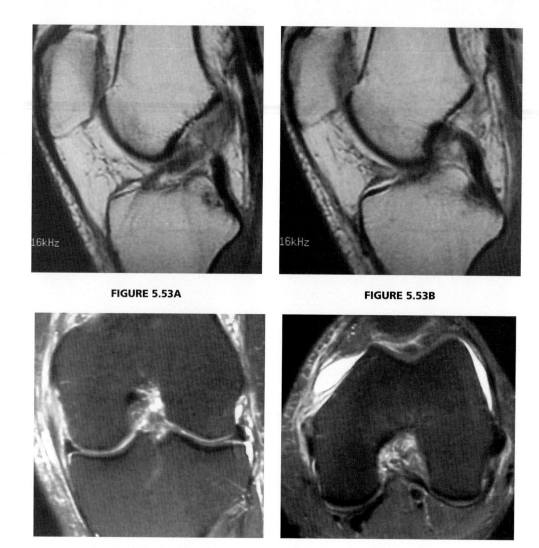

FIGURE 5.53A

FIGURE 5.53B

FIGURE 5.53C

FIGURE 5.53D

CLINICAL HISTORY

Knee pain and positive anterior drawer sign after injury.

FINDINGS

On the sagittal proton-density images (Fig. 5.53A–B), the anterior cruciate ligament (ACL) fibers are disrupted in the midsubstance of the ligament. The posterior cruciate ligament (PCL) is slightly bowed (Fig. 5.53B). The coronal and axial fat-suppressed proton-density images show a joint effusion and absence of the normal dark signal band of the ACL adjacent to the inner aspect of the lateral femoral condyle (Fig. 5.53C–D). The coronal image also shows edema around the medial collateral ligament (MCL) and high signal within the proximal fibers of the MCL (Fig. 5.53C).

DIAGNOSIS

Complete tear of the anterior cruciate ligament and partial tear of the medial collateral ligament.

DISCUSSION

The ACL arises posteromedially from the inner aspect of the lateral femoral condyle and passes inferiorly and anterolaterally to insert anterior and lateral to the anterior tibial spine. It is an extrasynovial but intraarticular fan-shaped ligament with its broader and stronger insertion on the tibia (1). The ACL is an important knee stabilizer, preventing anterior displacement and rotation of the tibia with respect to the femur, particularly with internal rotation and full extension of the knee (2).

The ACL is frequently injured during sports, falls, and motor vehicle accidents (3). The mechanism of ACL injury is complex, typically due to a combination of deceleration, hyperextension, and internal rotation. Tears of the ACL can be isolated or, more commonly, associated with additional ligamentous, meniscal, or bone injuries (4–6). Common associated injuries include tears of the MCL and medial meniscus (the O'Donoghue's triad) (4), tears of the posterior horn of the lateral meniscus, posterolateral tibial plateau fractures, and lateral femoral condyle contusions (5,6). Symptoms include pain and swelling as well as a subjective sensation of instability. Clinical evaluation of ACL injury includes stress testing such as the anterior drawer sign, the Lachman sign, and the Pivot Shift test (3).

Accurate MR imaging evaluation of ACL tears requires all three imaging planes (7). In the oblique sagittal plane, the middle and distal portions of the ACL are best seen. The proximal fibers of the ACL are often seen to better advantage on the coronal and axial images, appearing as a homogeneous low-signal band adjacent to the lateral femoral condyle (2).

The sensitivity and specificity of MR for the diagnosis of ACL injury is high (greater than 93%) (7). The primary sign of a tear of the ACL is discontinuity or nonvisualization of the ACL. Focal edema within the ACL is typically present in an acute injury. On the sagittal images, the torn distal ACL fibers become more horizontal than the Blumensaat line (roof of the intercondylar notch). In chronic ACL injury, the ligament is often lax and curved, and its scarred fibers appear thickened. Indirect signs of ACL tears include buckling of the PCL, anterior translocation of the tibia, and osseous and cartilage abnormalities. Fracture of the lateral tibial (Segond fracture), marrow edema in the lateral femoral condyle, posterolateral or posteromedial tibial plateau (8,9), and deepening of the lateral femoral notch greater than 2 mm are suggestive of ACL tears (10,11).

REFERENCES

1. Resnick D. Knee. In: Resnick D, Kang HS, eds. *Internal derangements of joints.* Philadelphia: WB Saunders, 1997:679–691.
2. Remer EM, Fitzgerald SW, Friedman H, et al. Anterior cruciate ligament injury: MR imaging diagnosis and patterns of injury. *Radiographics* 1992;12:901–915.
3. Yahey TN, Meyer SF, Shelbourne KD, et al. MR imaging of anterior cruciate ligament injuries. *Magn Reson Imaging Clin N Am* 1994;2:365–380.
4. Staron RB, Haramati N, Feldman F, et al. O'Donoghue's triad MRI evidence. *Skeletal Radiol* 1994;23:633–636.
5. Stallenberg B, Gevenois PA, Sintzoff JSA, et al. Fracture of the posterior aspect of the lateral tibial plateau: radiographic sign of anterior cruciate ligament tear. *Radiology* 1993;187:821–825.
6. Kaplan PA, Walker CW, Kilcoyne RF, et al. Occult fracture patterns of the knee associated with anterior cruciate ligament tears: assessment with MR imaging. *Radiology* 1992;183:835–838.
7. Fitzgerald SW, Remer EM, Friedman H, et al. MR evaluation of the anterior cruciate ligament: value of supplementing sagittal images with coronal and axial images. *AJR* 1993;160:1233–1237.
8. Kaplan PA, Gehl RH, Dussault RG, et al. Bone contusions of the posterior lip of the medial tibial plateau (contrecoup injury) and associated internal derangements of the knee at MR imaging. *Radiology* 1999;211:747–753.
9. Chan KK, Resnick D, Goodwin D, et al. Posteromedial tibial plateau injury including avulsion fracture of the semimembranous tendon insertion site: ancillary sign of anterior cruciate ligament tear at MR imaging. *Radiology* 1999;211:754–758.
10. Gentili A, Seeger LL, Yao L, et al. Anterior cruciate ligament tear: indirect signs at MR imaging. *Radiology* 1994;193:835–840.
11. Robertson PL, Schweitzer ME, Bartolozzi AR, et al. Anterior cruciate ligament tears: evaluation of multiple signs with MR imaging. *Radiology* 1994;193:829–834.

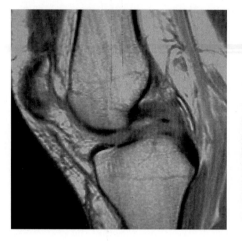

FIGURE 5.54A

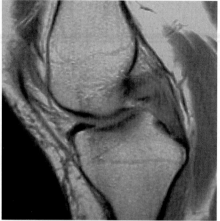

FIGURE 5.54B

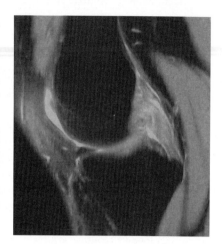

FIGURE 5.54C

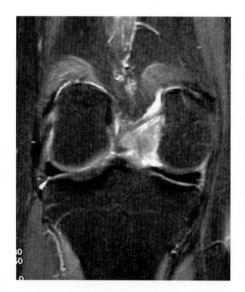

FIGURE 5.54D

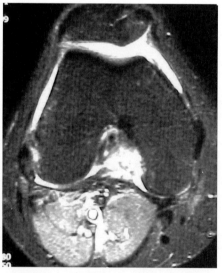

FIGURE 5.54E

CLINICAL HISTORY

A 28-year-old female with knee pain for 3 months following a motor vehicle accident.

FINDINGS

On sagittal proton-density (Fig. 5.54A) and coronal T1-weighted (Fig. 5.54B) images, amorphous increased signal intensity is present in the midportion of the posterior cruciate ligament (PCL), replacing the normal dark band of fibers (Fig. 5.54A–B). On the short tau inversion recovery (STIR) (Fig. 5.54C) and fat-suppressed proton-density (Fig. 5.54D–E) sequences, increased signal is seen within and surrounding the PCL (Fig. 5.54C–E). The tibia is subluxed posteriorly relative to the femur (Fig. 5.54A–C).

DIAGNOSIS

Complete tear of the posterior cruciate ligament.

DISCUSSION

The PCL arises from the inner aspect of the medial femoral condyle and courses posteriorly, inferiorly, and medially to insert onto the posterior intercondylar fossa, just below the articular surface of the tibia (1,2). It is composed of multiple fiber bundles, divided into anterolateral and posteromedial portions. Like the ACL, the PCL is intraarticular but extrasynovial in structure and is surrounded by a synovial sheath reflected from the posterior capsule. The primary function of the PCL is to restrict posterior displacement and external rotation of the tibia.

The PCL is torn less frequently than the ACL, and the injury is more difficult to diagnose on clinical examination. The most common site of tear is in the midsubstance of the ligament. The PCL is typically injured because of either a direct blow to the flexed knee or knee hyperextension. Injury of the PCL due to a direct blow to the proximal anterior tibia is often due to impact of the knee against the dashboard during a motor vehicle accident, forcing the tibia to displace posteriorly. Hyperextension injury, or severe abduction or adduction with rotation, is typically due to sports injury (2,3). Associated injuries about the knee include tears of the ACL, medial collateral ligament, and lateral collateral ligament; meniscal tears; joint effusion; and bone bruise, which is typically located in the anterior aspect of the tibia (4). Isolated PCL tears are often managed conservatively.

On MR imaging, the normal PCL appears as an arcuate low-signal structure that is well visualized on all planes, though its entire course is best seen on the sagittal images. In a complete tear of the PCL, the dark fibrous band is thickened and replaced by amorphous areas of intermediate signal intensity on T1-weighted sequences and high signal intensity on T2-weighted sequences. Focal disruption and discontinuity of the fibers are also present, typically in the middle of the ligament. In the acute setting, hemorrhage or fluid collects within and around the ligament. In a partial tear of the PCL, abnormal signal intensity is present within the ligament but some portions of the ligament remain intact (4).

REFERENCES

1. Kennedy JC. The posterior cruciate ligament. *J Trauma* 1967;7:367–377.
2. Covey DC, Spapega AA. Current concepts review injuries of the posterior cruciate ligament. *J Bone Joint Surg [Am]* 1993;75:1376–1386.
3. Sonin AH, Fitzgerald SW, Hoff FL, et al. MR imaging of the posterior cruciate ligament: normal, abnormal, and associated injury patterns. *Radiographics* 1995;15:551–561.
4. Sonin AH, Fitzgerald SW, Friedman H, et al. Posterior cruciate ligament injury: MR imaging diagnosis and patterns of injury. *Radiology* 1994;190:455–458.

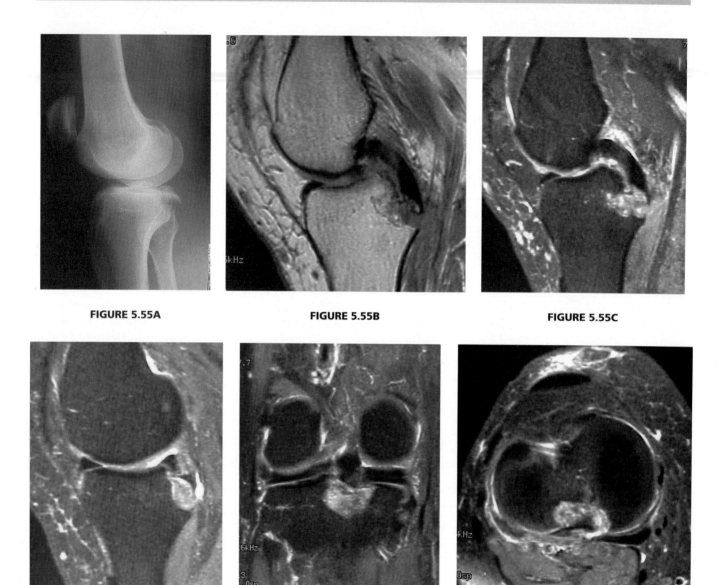

FIGURE 5.55A

FIGURE 5.55B

FIGURE 5.55C

FIGURE 5.55D

FIGURE 5.55E

FIGURE 5.55F

CLINICAL HISTORY

A 77-year-old female injured her knee 3 months ago and complained of persistent knee pain.

FINDINGS

The lateral radiograph (Fig. 5.55A) shows an avulsion fracture of the posterior tibia at the site of attachment of the posterior cruciate ligament (PCL). On the sagittal MR images (Fig. 5.55B–D), cortical disruption and abnormal signal intensity are present in the bone marrow at the posterior central portion of the tibia. A small bony fragment is dis-placed superiorly away from the tibial cortex (Fig. 5.55D) at the area of the PCL attachment site, but the ligament itself is intact. Increased signal intensity in the subchondral marrow at the avulsion fracture is also seen on the coronal (Fig. 5.55E) and axial (Fig. 5.55F) fat-suppressed T2-weighted fast spin-echo images.

DIAGNOSIS

Avulsion fracture at the tibial attachment of the posterior cruciate ligament.

DISCUSSION

The bony attachment of the PCL can be avulsed at either its femoral or tibial attachment site with sparing of the ligament itself (1–3). Avulsion fracture at the tibial attachment site is more common. The fracture can usually be seen on the lateral radiograph, where the normal oblique cortical bone of the PCL attachment site on the tibia, which normally is seen below the level of the tibial plateau, is displaced superiorly. The common mechanisms for this injury, either posterior tibial displacement in knee flexion or hyperextension, are identical to those causing ligament injury of the PCL. Although an isolated tear of the ligament itself is often managed conservatively, surgical reattachment of the avulsion fracture site is recommended (4).

REFERENCES

1. Mayer PJ, Micheli LJ. Avulsion of the femoral attachment of the posterior cruciate ligament in an eleven-year-old boy. Case report. *J Bone Joint Surg [Am]* 1979;61:431–432.
2. Torisu T. Isolated avulsion fracture of the tibial attachment of the posterior cruciate ligament. *J Bone Joint Surg [Am]* 1977;59:68–72.
3. Torisu T. Avulsion fracture of the tibial attachment of the posterior cruciate ligament: indications and results of delayed repair. *Clin Orthop* 1979; Sep(143):107–114.
4. Covey DC, Spapega AA. Current concepts review injuries of the posterior cruciate ligament. *J Bone Joint Surg [Am]* 1993;75:1376–1386.

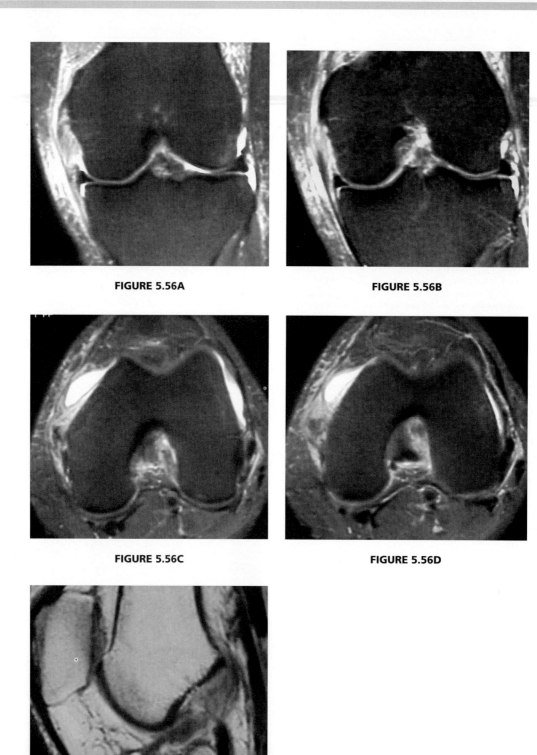

FIGURE 5.56A

FIGURE 5.56B

FIGURE 5.56C

FIGURE 5.56D

FIGURE 5.56E

CLINICAL HISTORY

A 20-year-old male complained of medial knee pain following a sports-related injury.

FINDINGS

On the coronal (Fig. 5.56A–B) and axial (Fig. 5.56C–D) fat-suppressed proton-density fast spin-echo images, irregularity, thickening, and high signal are noted within the medial collateral ligament (MCL). Increased signal is present within both the superficial (Fig. 5.56A) and deep fibers (Fig. 5.56B), and the proximal MCL fibers are undulating and irregular. There is extensive soft-tissue edema surrounding the MCL ligament as well as a moderate joint effusion.

High signal is also noted in the intercondylar notch, adjacent to the inner surface of the lateral femoral condyle (Fig. 5.56D). On the sagittal proton-density-weighted image Fig. 5.56E), the dark band of the anterior cruciate ligament (ACL) fibers is disrupted due to an associated complete tear of the ACL.

DIAGNOSIS

Tear of the medial collateral ligament and anterior cruciate ligaments.

DISCUSSION

The MCL arises from the medial epicondyle of the femur and inserts on the medial aspect of the proximal metaphysis of the tibia. The ligament has deep and superficial layers, which are separated by the thin, vertically oriented tibial collateral bursa. The intermediate-signal deep portion extends from the femur to the middle portion of the peripheral margin of the meniscus and tibia and is part of the true capsule of the knee (1). The low-signal superficial component is easier to see on MR and has a longer vertical extent, extending inferiorly to insert 5 to 7 cm below the joint line. The MCL is part of the medial supporting structures of the knee, restraining valgus angulation and rotation of the tibia and to some extent preventing anterior translation of the tibia.

On MR imaging, the MCL is best seen on coronal images at the middle portion of the knee, where the femur is widest. The normal MCL is a continuous low-signal-intensity band extending from the medial epicondyle of the femur to the metaphysis of the tibia. Thin linear regions of intermediate signal can be seen within the ligament due to fat surrounding the intraligamentous bursa.

Injury to the MCL has been classified into three grades based on the severity of the injury (2,3). Grade 1 injury represents strain of the MCL. On MR imaging, there is edema and hemorrhage in the soft tissues adjacent to the MCL but the ligament's fibers are intact. A grade 2 injury is a partial tear of the ligament. Some of the MCL fibers are disrupted and irregular, and there is abnormal high signal around and within the fibers but some intact fibers remain. The ligament may displace away from the adjacent bone. The grade 3 injury represents a complete tear with complete discontinuity of all the MCL fibers (4,5). Injuries of the MCL may be isolated or associated with additional injuries, including meniscal tear, meniscocapsular separation, ACL tear, and tibial or femoral bone bruises (4,6,7).

REFERENCES

1. Warren LF, Marshall JL. The supporting structures and layers on the medial side of the knee: an anatomical analysis. *J Bone Joint Surg [Am]* 1979;61:56–62.
2. Rasenberg EI, Lemmens JA, van Kampen A, et al. Grading medial collateral ligament injury: comparison of MR imaging and instrumented valgus-varus laxity test-device. A prospective double-blind patient study. *Eur J Radiol* 1995;21:18–24.
3. Yao L, Dungan D, Seeger LL. MR imaging of tibial collateral ligament injury: comparison with clinical examination. *Skeletal Radiol* 1994;23:521–524.
4. Garvin GJ, Munk PL, Vellet AD. Tears of the medial collateral ligament: magnetic resonance imaging findings and associated injuries. *Can Assoc Radiol J* 1993;44:199–204.
5. Resnick D. Knee. In: Resnick D, Kang HS, eds. *Internal derangements of joints.* Philadelphia: WB Saunders, 1997:639–642.
6. Hillard-Sembell D, Daniel DM, Stone ML, et al. Combined injuries of the anterior cruciate and medial collateral ligaments of the knee: effect of treatment on stability and function of the joint. *J Bone Joint Surg [Am]* 1996;78:169–176.
7. De Maeseneer M, Lenchik L, Starok M, et al. Normal and abnormal medial meniscocapsular structures: MR imaging and sonography in cadavers. *AJR* 1998;171:969–976.

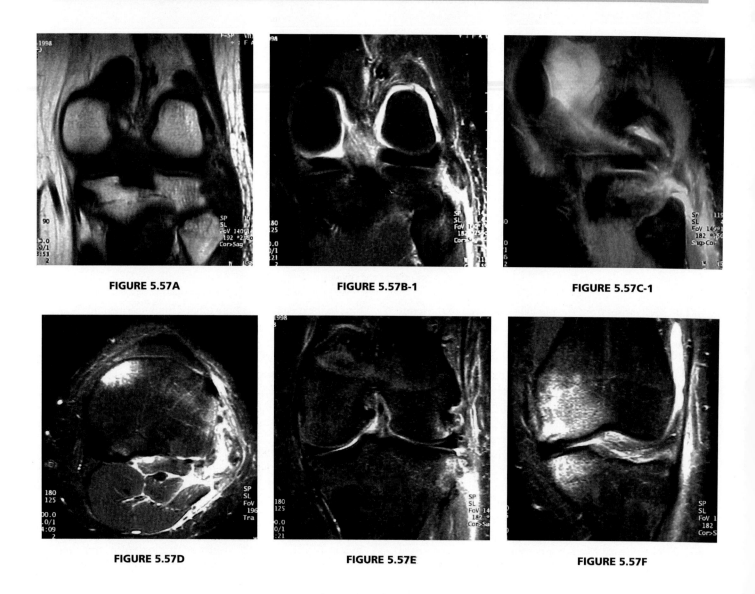

FIGURE 5.57A

FIGURE 5.57B-1

FIGURE 5.57C-1

FIGURE 5.57D

FIGURE 5.57E

FIGURE 5.57F

CLINICAL HISTORY

A 19-year-old male with lateral knee pain sustained a soccer injury 2 weeks prior to this MR examination.

FINDINGS

Coronal T1-weighted (Fig. 5.57A) and T2-weighted (Fig. 5.57B-1) images show disruption of the normal dark band of the lateral collateral ligament (LCL) (Fig. 5.57B-2, *arrow*) and biceps femoris tendons (Fig. 5.57B-2, *arrowhead*), which are absent and replaced with increased signal intensity. On the sagittal image, the normal V-shaped configuration formed by the LCL and biceps femoris tendon is also absent (Fig. 5.57C-2, *arrow*). Ligament disruption and extensive soft-tissue edema are present in the posterolateral soft tissues of the knee on the axial fat-suppressed proton-density image (Fig. 5.57D). The most posterior aspect of the iliotibial tract is irregular with increased signal around it (Fig. 5.57E). Bone marrow edema is present within the lateral portion of the lateral femoral condyle and proximal tibia. More anteriorly, extensive bone marrow edema is noted in the medial femoral condyle and medial tibial plateau (Fig. 5.57F).

DIAGNOSIS

Injury of the posterolateral corner of the knee with disruption of the lateral collateral ligament, biceps femoris tendon, and partial tear of the iliotibial tract.

DISCUSSION

The lateral supporting structures of the knee are stronger than those on the medial side and are therefore injured less frequently. The anatomy of the lateral capsular structures of the knee is complex and has been depicted in various ways (1–4). Typically, the lateral supporting structures are grouped into three layers (1–3). The main structures in the superficial layer are the iliotibial tract and portions of the biceps femoris tendon. The second layer, which lies deep to the superficial layer, consists of the lateral patellar retinaculum and the patellofemoral ligament (5). The third layer, which is the deepest layer, includes the lateral collateral ligament, the fabellofibular ligament, and the arcuate ligament (1). The lateral capsule prevents varus angulation and external rotation of the knee (5). Excessive knee hyperextension, external rotation, and varus angulation can injure the LCL and related posterolateral supporting structures, leading to instability.

On MR imaging, the normal LCL and biceps femoris can be identified as dark bands on sagittal, coronal, and axial images. The LCL arises from the lateral epicondyle of the femur and courses posteriorly and inferiorly to insert onto the proximal lateral surface of the fibular head, along with the biceps femoris tendon. Where the LCL and biceps femoris tendon merge forms a V-shaped structure on the peripheral sagittal images. MR imaging is an excellent technique for assessment of posterolateral knee injury and allows preoperative planning of repair of this complex region (6). Associated injuries of other supporting structures such as the arcuate ligament, popliteus tendon, and iliotibial tract can also be readily identified with MR imaging.

Like the medial collateral ligament, LCL injury is divided into three grades, depending on the severity of the injury (7). Severe injuries result in considerable instability and allow abnormal knee motion. When the posterolateral structures are torn, the anteromedial femoral condyle impacts upon the tibia, producing a characteristic bone contusion pattern, with edema at the anteromedial femoral condyle and at the anteromedial tibial plateau (6). This typical contusion pattern is evident in this case.

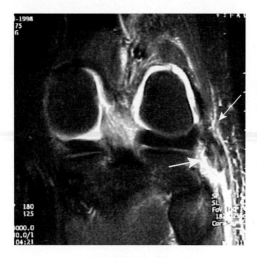
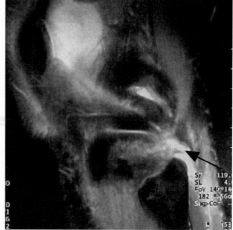

FIGURE 5.57B-2   **FIGURE 5.57C-2**

REFERENCES

1. Seebacher JR, Inglis AE, Marshall JL, et al. The structure of the posterolateral aspect of the knee. *J Bone Joint Surg [Am]* 1982;64:536–541.
2. Terry GC, LaPrade RF. The posterolateral aspect of the knee: anatomy and surgical approach. *Am J Sports Med* 1996;24:732–739.
3. Kim YC, Chung IH, Yoo WK, et al. Anatomy and magnetic resonance imaging of the posterolateral structures of the knee. *Clin Anat* 1997;10:397–404.
4. Ruiz ME, Erickson SJ. Medial and lateral supporting structures of the knee: normal MR imaging anatomy and pathologic findings. *Magn Reson Imaging Clin N Am* 1994;2:381–399.
5. Resnick D. Knee. In: Resnick D, Kang HS, eds. *Internal derangements of joints.* Philadelphia: WB Saunders, 1997:647–653.
6. Ross G, Chapman AW, Newberg AR, et al. Magnetic resonance imaging for the evaluation of acute posterolateral complex injuries of the knee. *Am J Sports Med* 1997;25:444–448.
7. Mirowitz SA, Shu HH. MR imaging evaluation of knee collateral ligaments and related injuries: comparison of T1-weighted, T2-weighted, and fat-saturated T2-weighted sequences—correlation with clinical findings. *J Magn Reson Imaging* 1994;4:725–732.

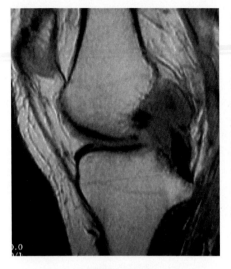

FIGURE 5.58A

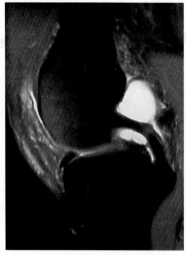

FIGURE 5.58B

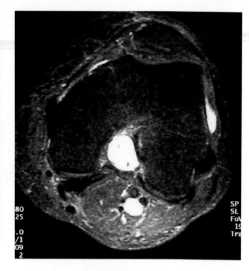

FIGURE 5.58C

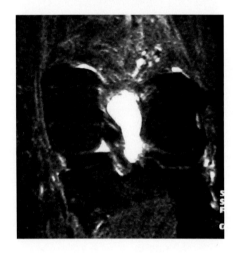

FIGURE 5.58D

CLINICAL HISTORY

A 57-year-old male complained of chronic knee pain.

FINDINGS

Sagittal T1-weighted (Fig. 5.58A) and sagittal fat-suppressed proton-density-weighted images (Fig. 5.58B) show a well-defined, homogeneous mass surrounding the posterior cruciate ligament (PCL) in the intercondylar fossa, The mass is located near the femoral attachment site of the PCL. The mass has a few very thin septae within it and shows signal characteristics consistent with fluid appearances. The PCL and the anterior cruciate ligament (ACL) are both intact, but the cruciate ligaments are distorted and compressed by the lesion. Note the compression of the ACL against the inner aspect of the femoral condyle (Fig. 5.58C). There is also small pressure erosion of the inner aspect of the lateral femoral condyle (Fig. 5.58D).

DIAGNOSIS

Intraarticular ganglion cyst arising from the posterior cruciate ligament.

DISCUSSION

Intraarticular ganglion cysts of the knee are uncommon benign fluid collections that typically arise from the alar folds that cover either the infrapatellar fat pad or the cruciate ligaments (1). The etiology of intraarticular ganglion cysts is unclear, but they are thought to be acquired lesions (2). Most ganglia are clinically asymptomatic, though symptoms of pain and swelling may be present, depending on the location and size of the cyst. When the ganglion cyst is located around a cruciate ligament, restricted extension or flexion of the knee may develop (2,3).

On MR imaging, a ganglion cyst appears as a well-circumscribed mass with internal signal characteristic of fluid. A thin, low-signal, fibrous capsule or thin internal septations may be seen (4). Ganglion cysts that arise from the ACL may have a fusiform appearance, extending along the surface of the ACL or interspersed within its fibers. Cysts arising from the PCL are usually well defined and multiloculated, and rarely communicate with the joint (5). Their location is variable, but they commonly form at either the femoral or tibial insertion of the PCL (2).

The major differential diagnostic consideration is a pericruciate meniscal cyst associated with a tear of the posterior horn of the medial meniscus (6) (Fig. 5.12E–F). A meniscal cyst is associated with a tear of the posterior horn of the medial meniscus, whereas a true PCL ganglion cyst is not associated with meniscal pathology. Meniscal cysts often show a communicating channel between the cyst and the torn meniscus. Meniscal cysts typically extending cranially from their posteroinferior origin are located posterior to the PCL. PCL ganglion cysts may arise from either the femoral or tibial insertion sites of the PCL.

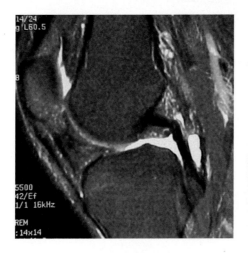

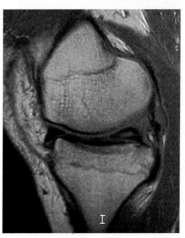

FIGURE 5.58E   **FIGURE 5.58F**

REFERENCES

1. Resnick D. Knee. In: Resnick D, Kang HS, eds. *Internal derangements of joints.* Philadelphia: WB Saunders, 1997:582–589.
2. Bui-Mansfield LT, Youngberg RA. Intraarticular ganglia of the knee: prevalence, presentation, etiology, and management. *AJR* 1997;168:123–127.
3. Steiner E, Steinbach LS, Schnarkowski P, et al. Ganglia and cysts around joints. *Radiol Clin North Am* 1996;34:395–425.
4. Nokes SR, Koonce TW. Ganglion cysts of the cruciate ligaments of the knee: recognition on MR images and CT-guided aspiration. *AJR* 1994;162:1504.
5. Recht MP, Applegate G, Kaplan P, et al. The MR appearance of cruciate ganglion cysts: a report of 16 cases. *Skeletal Radiol* 1994;23:597–600.
6. Lektrakul N, Skaf A, Yeh LR, et al. Pericruciate meniscal cysts arising from tear of the posterior horn of the medial meniscus: MR imaging features that simulate posterior cruciate ganglion cysts. *AJR* 1999;172:1575–1579.

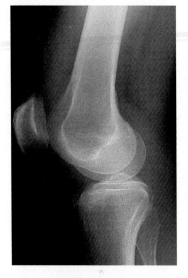

FIGURE 5.59A

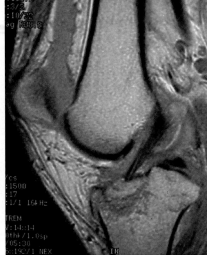

FIGURE 5.59B

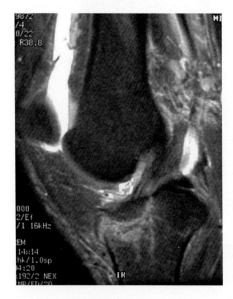

FIGURE 5.59C

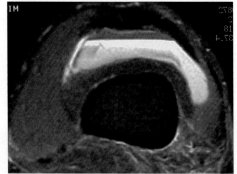

FIGURE 5.59D

CLINICAL HISTORY

A 41-year-old man presented with persistent knee pain and swelling after an injury.

FINDINGS

The lateral radiograph shows a large joint effusion with a fat-fluid level (Fig. 5.59A). There is subtle cortical irregularity of the anterior tibia just below the joint line. Sagittal proton-density, and sagittal and axial fat-suppressed proton-density images demonstrate a large joint effusion with three layers of fluid within the joint (Fig. 5.59B–D). The most superior layer has signal characteristics diagnostic of fat. The middle layer is high signal intensity on the proton-density-weighted images and is due to serum. The most inferior layer shows relatively low signal due to layering of blood cells and hemosiderin.

Abnormal linear lines of low signal intensity, with surrounding marrow edema, are present in the anterior tibial plateau (Fig. 5.59B–C). The anterior and superior tibial cortexes are disrupted at the base of the anterior cruciate ligament. These linear densities are due to an undisplaced fracture of the tibial eminence.

DIAGNOSIS

Acute fracture of the tibial eminence with associated lipohemarthrosis.

DISCUSSION

Nondisplaced fractures can be difficult to detect on conventional radiography, but the presence of lipohemarthrosis is strongly suggestive of an osseous injury. MR imaging is very sensitive for the diagnosis of subtle fractures or bone bruises and has replaced scintigraphy and computed tomography for the diagnosis of radiographically occult bone trauma. Advantages of MR imaging include concomitant evaluation of associated meniscal and ligamentous injuries (1).

In adults, occult fractures of the knee occur most commonly at the tibial plateau, with lateral tibial plateau fractures being more common than those involving the medial plateau (2). Avulsion fractures of the intercondylar eminence and tibial spines can also be difficult to identify on conventional radiographs, as in this case. Fractures of the tibial spine or intercondylar eminence are caused by twisting, abduction-adduction, or impaction with the femoral condyle (3).

Very often these types of injuries are associated with a tear of the anterior cruciate ligament and the menisci (4). An avulsion fracture of the anterior tibial eminence directly at the anterior cruciate attachment site, as seen in this example, is most common in children and young adolescents.

On MR imaging, STIR- and T1-weighted sequences are usually best for diagnosis of osseous fractures (5). The fracture lines themselves are low in signal intensity on all imaging sequences. On STIR- and T2-weighted images, the edema surrounding the fracture is bright, whereas the edematous bone is low signal on the T1-weighted images. Large amounts of bone marrow can sometimes obscure the fracture lines themselves, particularly on STIR images (5). In general, bone marrow edema is more prominent when the fracture is due to impaction rather than avulsion (3). In this patient, the fracture is most likely avulsive in nature because of the minimal edema surrounding the fractures.

REFERENCES

1. Barrow BA, Fajman WA, Parker LM, et al. Tibial plateau fractures: evaluation with MR imaging. *Radiographics* 1994;14:553–559.
2. Hohl M. Tibial condylar fractures. *J Bone Joint Surg* 1067;49:1455–1467.
3. Resnick D. Knee. In: Resnick D, Kang HS, eds. *Internal derangements of joints.* Philadelphia: WB Saunders, 1997:567–570.
4. Kendall NS, Hsu SY, Chan K-M. Fracture of the tibial spine in adults and children: a review of 31 cases. *J Bone Joint Surg* 1992;74:848.
5. Meyers SP, Wiener SN. Magnetic resonance imaging features of fractures using the short tau inversion recovery (STIR) sequence: correlation with radiographic findings. *Skeletal Radiol* 1991;20:499–507.

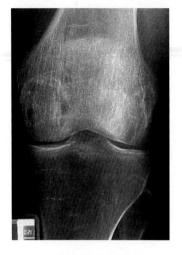

FIGURE 5.60A

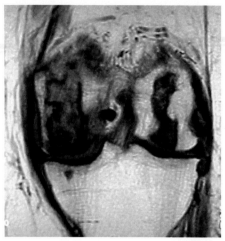

FIGURE 5.60B

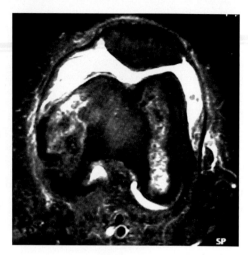

FIGURE 5.60C

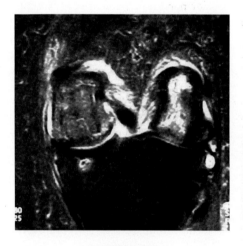

FIGURE 5.60D

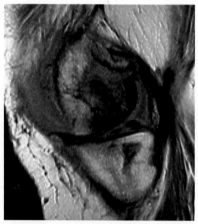

FIGURE 5.60E

CLINICAL HISTORY

A 73-year-old woman complained of chronic atraumatic knee pain. She had taken corticosteroids for several years for chronic obstructive lung disease.

FINDINGS

The frontal radiograph of the knee (Fig. 5.60A) shows patchy sclerosis in both femoral condyles and minimal flattening of the medial femoral condyle. The coronal T1-weighted (Fig. 5.60B), coronal and axial STIR (Fig. 5.60C–D), and sagittal proton-density-weighted (Fig. 5.60E) images show well-circumscribed lesions in both femoral condyles, as well as a small lesion in the medial tibial plateau. These lesions abut the subchondral bone and show serpinginous low-signal-intensity margins that surround areas of heterogeneous signal marrow. Within the femoral lesions, intermixed regions of marrow edema and fat signal are identified. There is an effusion, mild soft-tissue edema, and changes of osteoarthritis. The sagittal proton-density-weighted image also illustrates linear high signal within the posterior horn of the medial meniscus that extends to the inferior articulating surface.

DIAGNOSIS

Avascular necrosis of both femoral condyles and medial tibial plateau. Tear of the posterior horn of the medial meniscus.

DISCUSSION

Avascular necrosis, also known as osteonecrosis, refers to the death of both trabecular bone and bone marrow elements (1). In an attempt to repair the necrotic bone, remodeling by resorption of the necrotic material and deposition of new bone takes place. During this process, weight-bearing bone becomes mechanically weakened and may eventually collapse, leading secondarily to osteoarthritis and debilitating pain (2). There are many causes of osteonecrosis and the knee is commonly involved, particularly the femoral condyles (3). Some common causes of osteonecrosis include posttraumatic vascular disruption, alcoholism, corticosteroid therapy, Cushing's disease, the hemoglobinopathies (e.g., sickle cell disease), collagen vascular disorders (e.g., systemic lupus erythematosus and rheumatoid arthritis), and irradiation (3).

MR imaging is the most sensitive modality for early diagnosis of this condition. MR findings vary according to the stage of osteonecrosis. In the early stages of osteonecrosis, the area of infarction shows ill-defined regions of bone marrow edema that are intermediate to low signal intensity on T1-weighted sequences and high signal intensity on T2-weighted sequences. In later stages, infarcts typically are well marginated by a serpentine band or ring of low signal intensity on both T1- and T2-weighted images. This serpentine zone of low signal intensity, representing bone sclerosis or fibrosis at the margin of the infarct, surrounds a necrotic region with variable signal intensity. Within the infarcted area, small areas of fatty marrow signal intensity can often be identified, differentiating infarcts from neoplasms, which rarely contain fat signal within the lesion (3,4). In more advanced stages, subchondral fractures and cortical collapse of the weight-bearing articular surface can be seen. The size of the area of infarction is an important prognostic feature. Larger infarcts, particularly those involving the weight-bearing surface, show a higher tendency to undergo collapse (5).

REFERENCES

1. Bluemke DA, Zerhouni EA. MRI of avascular necrosis of bone. *Top Magn Reson Imaging* 1996;8:231–246.
2. Ahuja SC, Bullough PG. Osteonecrosis of the knee: a clinicopathological study in twenty-eight patients. *J Bone Joint Surg [Am]* 1978;60:191–197.
3. Resnick D, Niwayama G. Osteonecrosis: pathogenesis. In: Resnick D, Niwayama G, eds. *Diagnosis of bone and joint disorders*, 3rd ed. Philadelphia: WB Saunders, 1996:Chapter 79.
4. Kubo T, Yamazoe S, Sugano N, et al. Initial MRI findings of nontraumatic osteonecrosis of the femoral head in renal allograft recipients. *Magn Reson Imaging* 1997;15:1017–1023.
5. Sakai T, Sugano N, Ohzono K, et al. MRI evaluation of steroid- or alcohol-related osteonecrosis of the femoral condyle. *Acta Orthop Scand* 1998;69:598–602.

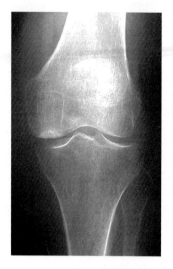

FIGURE 5.61A

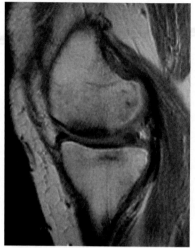

FIGURE 5.61B

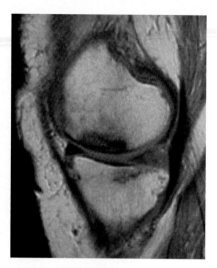

FIGURE 5.61C-1

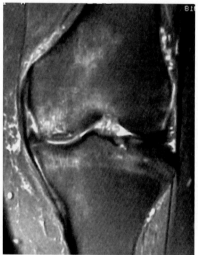

FIGURE 5.61D

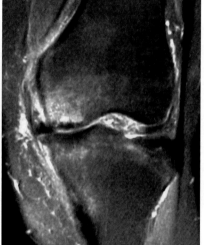

FIGURE 5.61E

CLINICAL HISTORY

A 70-year-old female complained of the abrupt onset of severe knee pain.

FINDINGS

The anteroposterior radiograph of the knee (Fig. 5.61A) shows osteopenia and a semilunar area of focal sclerosis on the weight-bearing surface of the medial femoral condyle. Sagittal proton-density-weighted images (Fig. 5.61B–C-1) demonstrate an irregular region of low signal intensity in the subchondral bone of the medial femoral condyle that is marginated posteriorly by a low-signal line (Fig. 5.61C-2, *arrow*). A similar but shorter line of low signal is present in the proximal tibial epiphysis.

The coronal fat-suppressed proton images (Fig. 5.61D–E) show diffuse marrow edema in the subchondral regions of the medial femur and tibia. Within the marrow edema, a linear low-signal line is noted in the subchondral bone of the femur, paralleling the articular surface. In the tibial epiphysis, an irregular band of high signal intensity is visible (Fig. 5.61D).

DIAGNOSIS

Spontaneous osteonecrosis of the medial femoral condyle. Presumed insufficiency fracture or small infarct of the proximal tibia.

DISCUSSION

Spontaneous or idiopathic osteonecrosis of the knee is a condition that affects predominantly middle-aged and elderly females. Typically, the patient complains of the sudden onset of severe knee pain without any antecedent trauma (1,2). The weight-bearing surface of the medial femoral condyle is most commonly involved. Other affected sites in the knee, in order of frequency, are the medial and lateral tibial plateaus, and the lateral femoral condyle. Although the etiology of spontaneous osteonecrosis remains unclear, the condition is thought to be due to vascular insufficiency of the subchondral bone, leading to infarction (1). For reasons that are unclear, this condition is frequently associated with underlying meniscal pathology and osteoarthritis.

Initial radiographs are usually normal. As the condition progresses, subchondral sclerosis develops, followed by subchondral lucency and flattening of the cortical surface (1). MR imaging is more sensitive than radiography for detecting early spontaneous osteonecrosis of the knee. In the early stages of osteonecrosis, only amorphous bone marrow edema is present, resulting in low-signal marrow on T1-weighted images and high signal intensity on T2-weighted or STIR sequences. In the elderly patient with degenerative joint disease, this MR appearance is rather nonspecific and difficult to distinguish from the edema that can be seen with advanced osteoarthritis. In later stages of osteonecrosis, low-signal lines are visible within the subchondral bone. The location of this low-signal line helps predict the outcome of the lesion. When the line is absent or very near the articular surface, the lesion may resolve spontaneously; when the line extends deeper into the marrow, the lesion tends to be irreversible (3). In advanced disease, subchondral collapse leads to flattening of the articular surface.

The diagnosis of spontaneous osteonecrosis of the knee requires exclusion of many known causes of ischemic necrosis of bone, such as chronic steroid use, renal transplantation, hemoglobinopathy, alcoholism, and underlying vasculitis (1). In elderly patients, similar changes in the subchondral bone have also been described following meniscectomy, particularly if there has been concomitant debridement of degenerated cartilage (4–6).

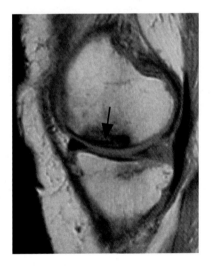

FIGURE 5.61C-2

REFERENCES

1. Resnick D, Niwayama G. Osteonecrosis: diagnostic technique, specific situations, and complications. In: Resnick D, Niwayama G, eds. *Diagnosis of bone and joint disorders*, 3rd ed. Philadelphia: WB Saunders, 1996:Chapter 80.
2. Williams JL, Cliff MM, Bonakdarpour A. Spontaneous osteonecrosis of the knee. *Radiology* 1973;107:15–19.
3. Lecouvet FE, Van de Berg BC, Maldague BE, et al. Early irreversible osteonecrosis versus transient lesions of the femoral condyles: prognostic value of subchondral bone and marrow changes on MR imaging. *AJR* 1998;170:71–77.
4. Prues-Latour V, Bonvin JC, Fritschy D. Nine cases of osteonecrosis in elderly patients following arthroscopic meniscectomy. *Knee Surg Sports Traumatol Arthrosc* 1998;6:142–147.
5. Rozbruch SR, Wickiewicz TL, DiCarlo EF, et al. Osteonecrosis of the knee following arthroscopic laser meniscectomy. *Arthroscopy* 1996;12:245–250.
6. Santori N, Condello V, Adriani E, et al. Osteonecrosis after arthroscopic medial meniscectomy. *Arthroscopy* 1995;11:220–224.

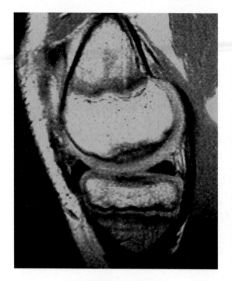

FIGURE 5.62A

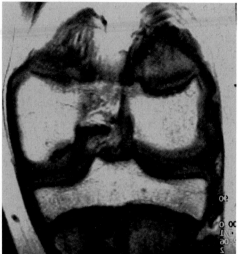

FIGURE 5.62B

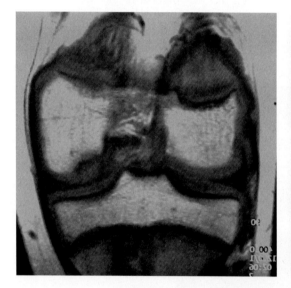

FIGURE 5.62C

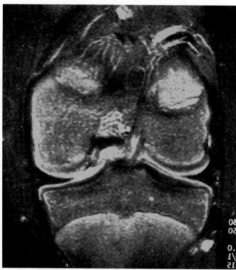

FIGURE 5.62D

CLINICAL HISTORY

This 14-year-old boy complained of medial knee pain.

FINDINGS

Sagittal proton-density (Fig. 5.62A) and coronal T1-weighted (Fig. 5.62B–C) images show a crescentic region of low signal intensity in the subchondral region of the inner aspect of the medial femoral condyle. On the coronal STIR sequence, this area shows minimal increased signal within this lesion (Fig. 5.62D). There is no fluid signal present between the low-signal abnormality and the parent bone and the cartilage appears intact.

DIAGNOSIS

Osteochondritis dissecans of the medial femoral condyle.

DISCUSSION

Osteochondritis dissecans (OCD) refers to fragmentation and potential separation of a portion of the subchondral bone and its overlying articular surface. OCD can occur at any joint, but its most common location is the femoral condyle, typically at the lateral portion of the medial femoral condyle (1,2). Although OCD is typically unilateral, it can occur bilaterally. The etiology of OCD remains unclear, but approximately half of affected patients have a history of preceding trauma (3).

Clinical presentation is usually during adolescence, with males affected more frequently than females. Typical symptoms of OCD include knee pain that is aggravated by motion, clicking, swelling, or locking, though small lesions may be asymptomatic (4). OCD can resolve spontaneously, especially in young children. If the lesion does progress and the chondral or osteochondral fragment undergoes separation from the parent bone, the resultant articular incongruity can lead to premature osteoarthritis.

MR is very accurate for evaluating the stage of OCD and the status of the overlying cartilage. The presence of high signal intensity between the lesion and the parent bone on T2-weighted sequences suggests granulation tissue or fluid at the interface and is considered a sign of instability of the lesion. The absence of such high signal generally indicates a stable lesion. Stable lesions and lesions that are smaller than 160 mm^2 have a relatively good outcome. Large size and instability portend an unfavorable outcome (5,6).

REFERENCES

1. Obedian RS, Grelsamer RP. Osteochondritis dissecans of the distal femur and patella. *Clin Sports Med* 1997;16:157–174.
2. Aichroth P. Osteochondritis dissecans of the knee: a clinical survey. *J Bone Joint Surg [Br]* 1971;53:440–447.
3. Mesgarzadeh M, Sapega AA, Bonakdarpour A, et al. Osteochondritis dissecans: analysis of mechanical stability with radiography, scintigraphy, and MR imaging. *Radiology* 1987;165:775–780.
4. Resnick D, Niwayama G. Osteonecrosis: pathogenesis. In: Resnick D, Niwayama G, eds. *Diagnosis of bone and joint disorders*, 3rd ed. Philadelphia: WB Saunders, 1996:Chapter 79.
5. De Smet AA, Ilahi OA, Graf BK. Untreated osteochondritis dissecans of the femoral condyles: prediction of patient outcome using radiographic and MR findings. *Skeletal Radiol* 1997;26:463–467.
6. De Smet AA, Ilahi OA, Graf BK. Reassessment of the MR criteria for stability of osteochondritis dissecans in the knee and ankle. *Skeletal Radiol* 1996;25:159–163.

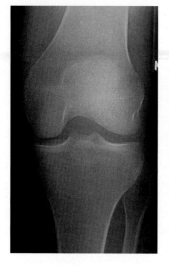

FIGURE 5.63A-1

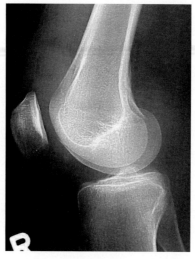

FIGURE 5.63B-1

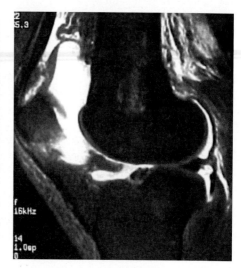

FIGURE 5.63C

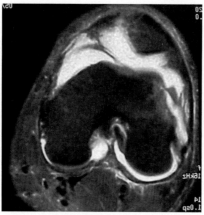

FIGURE 5.63D-1

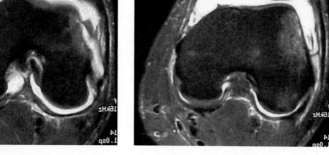

FIGURE 5.63E

CLINICAL HISTORY

A 31-year-old female acutely traumatized her knee.

FINDINGS

The radiographs (Fig. 5.63A-1, B-1) show slight flattening of the medial aspect of the patella (Fig. 5.63A-2, *arrow*) and a large joint effusion. A small bony fragment is present in the anterior joint space (Fig. 5.63B-2, *arrow*). On the sagittal and axial fat-suppressed T2-weighted images, the medial and inferior aspects of the patella appear irregular (Fig. 5.63C), and the patellar cartilage is fragmented (Fig. 5.63C and 5.63E). The fractured patellar fragment lies ad-

jacent to the lateral femoral condyle (Fig. 5.63D-2, *arrow*). Bone marrow edema is present within the anterolateral aspect of the lateral femoral condyle, and there is edema in the adjacent soft tissues (Fig. 5.63D–E). The medial patellar retinaculum (Fig. 5.63D-1 and 5.63E) is attenuated and partially disrupted with edema around it. There is lipohemarthrosis within the knee joint.

DIAGNOSIS

Spontaneously reduced lateral patellar dislocation with medial patellar fracture, lateral femoral condyle contusion, and disruption of the medial patellar retinaculum.

DISCUSSION

Patellar dislocation refers to the complete dislocation of the patella out of the trochlear sulcus of the distal femur. Lateral dislocation of the patella is far more common than medial dislocation. Other rare types of patellar dislocations include the vertical and rotational forms (1). Patellar dislocation represents 2% to 3% of all knee injuries (2). Common mechanisms of patellar dislocation are either twisting, with internal rotation of the femur and simultaneous contraction of the quadriceps muscle, or a direct blow to the outside of the knee (3). This injury occurs most commonly in teenagers and young adults (4). Predisposing factors include patella alta, a shallow trochlear sulcus, abnormal insertion of the patellar tendon, quadriceps muscle weakness or a tight lateral retinaculum, and patellar dysplasias (3).

Following acute traumatic dislocation of the patellofemoral joint, the patella very often spontaneously relocates and most patients are unaware of the dislocation. Physical examination is limited due to a swollen and painful knee, making it difficult to distinguish prior patellar dislocation from other serious knee injuries. More than 50% of transient patellar dislocations are missed at the time of initial clinical examination. MR imaging dramatically increases the accuracy of the diagnosis (2). There is a characteristic constellation of MR findings strongly suggestive of this injury that allows MR imaging to accurately diagnose prior acute lateral patellar dislocation, even when the patella has been reduced to near anatomic location.

When the patella is dislocated laterally, it is drawn anteriorly out of the trochlear groove and then displaces laterally to lie external to the lateral femoral condyle. The medial patellar facet impacts against the outer surface of the lateral femoral condyle, leading to fracture or contusion of these opposing bony surfaces. MR imaging shows osteochondral fractures or marrow edema involving the inferomedial patella and anterolateral femoral condyle. Small bony fragments arising from avulsion fractures of the medial patella can sometimes be within the joint. When the patella reduces back into the trochlear groove, the patella again impacts against the lateral femoral condyle, leading to further osteochondral injury. Injury to the medial retinaculum, which is under tension during the dislocation, ranges from sprain to complete disruption and can occur at its patellar insertion site, at its midportion, or within the vastus medialis muscle. Increased signal on T2-weighted images is present within and around the medial retinaculum with disruption of the fibers. Additionally, disruption of the capsule, medial collateral ligament, and anterior cruciate ligament may be present (4).

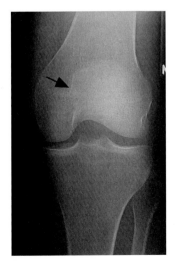

FIGURE 5.63A-2

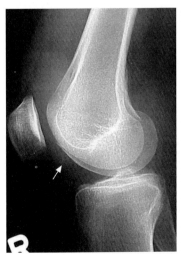

FIGURE 5.63B-2

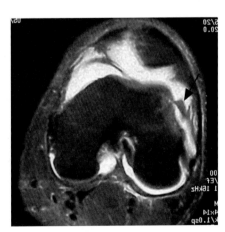

FIGURE 5.63D-2

REFERENCES

1. Resnick D, Kang HS. Knee. In: Resnick D, Kang HS, eds. *Internal derangements of joints.* Philadelphia: WB Saunders, 1997:706–707.
2. Kirsch MD, Fitzgerald SW, Friedman H, et al. Transient lateral patellar dislocation: diagnosis with MR imaging. *AJR* 1993;161:109–113.
3. Lance EA, Deutsch L, Mink JH. Prior lateral patellar dislocation: MR imaging findings. *Radiology* 1993;189:905–907.
4. Virolainen H, Visuri T, Kuusela T. Acute dislocation of the patella: MR findings. *Radiology* 1993;189:243–246.

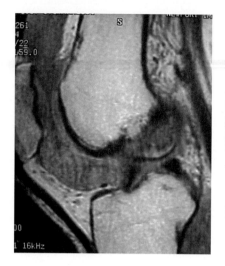

FIGURE 5.64A

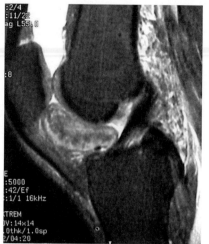

FIGURE 5.64B

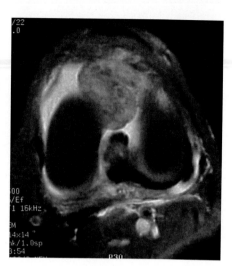

FIGURE 5.64C

CLINICAL HISTORY

A 32-year-old female with knee pain and swelling.

FINDINGS

Sagittal proton-density and T2-weighted images, and axial fat-suppressed proton-density-weighted images show a large effusion and an inhomogeneous, oval-shaped mass in the region of Hoffa's fat pad (Fig. 5.64A–C). In addition, irregular regions of inhomogeneous soft-tissue density are present in the posterior knee joint (Fig. 5.64B–C). These regions of soft-tissue proliferation are continuous with the synovial lining of the joint and heterogeneous in signal on all sequences. Within areas of synovial proliferation, there are multiple punctate areas that maintain low signal intensity on both the T2-weighted and the fat-suppressed proton-density-weighted sequences.

DIAGNOSIS

Pigmented villonodular synovitis.

DISCUSSION

Pigmented villonodular synovitis (PVNS) is a benign proliferative disorder of the synovium of unknown etiology (1). PVNS is almost always monoarticular, most commonly affecting the knee joint (2), followed by the hip, ankle, shoulder, and elbow articulations. Within the joint, PVNS can be diffuse or localized to a portion of the articulation. The localized form of PVNS is most common in the knee, where it appears as a well-defined mass within or posterior to Hoffa's fat pad, or in the posterior aspect of the joint (3). Young adults are most commonly affected, with a slight male predominance. Clinical signs and symptoms are nonspecific, including the insidious onset of swelling, pain, decreased range of motion, and a sensation of joint locking (4).

Conventional radiographs are often negative or reveal only a nonspecific effusion. Occasionally, radiographs show periarticular soft-tissue masses, erosive changes of the bone, or very rarely, calcification within the lesion. MR is an excellent tool for diagnosis and for determining the distribution and the extent of the disease (4,5). On MR imaging, the characteristic findings of PVNS are synovial proliferation, manifest as low signal on T1-weighted and intermediate signal on T2-weighted sequences. Within the areas of synovial hyperplasia, there are scattered foci that remain low signal on T2-weighted sequences, presumably due to hemosiderin deposition within and adjacent to the lesion (6,7). The areas of hemosiderin are most prominent on gradient-echo recalled sequences, where they enlarge and undergo blooming due to magnetic susceptibility artifacts. On STIR sequences, the lesion shows diffuse increased signal intensity throughout (1). After the intravenous administration of gadolinium, intense enhancement of the areas of PVNS is evident.

REFERENCES

1. Lin J, Jacobson JA, Jamadar DA, et al. Pigmented villonodular synovitis and related lesions: the spectrum of imaging findings. *AJR* 1999;172:191–197.
2. Hughes TH, Sartoris DJ, Schweitzer ME, et al. Pigmented villonodular synovitis: MRI characteristics. *Skeletal Radiol* 1995;24:7–12.
3. Bravo SM, Winalski CS, Weissman BN. Pigmented villonodular synovitis. *Radiol Clin North Am* 1996;34:311–326.
4. Mandelbaum BR, Grant TT, Hartzman S, et al. The use of MRI to assist in diagnosis of pigmented villonodular synovitis of the knee joint. *Clin Orthop* 1988;Jun(231):135–139.
5. Steinbach LS, Neumann CH, Stoller DW, et al. MRI of the knee in diffuse pigmented villonodular synovitis. *Clin Imaging* 1989;13:305–316.
6. Araki Y, Tanaka H, Yamamoto H, et al. MR imaging of pigmented villonodular synovitis of the knee. *Radiat Med* 1994;12:11–15.
7. Spritzer CE, Dalinka MK, Kressel HY. Magnetic resonance imaging of pigmented villonodular synovitis: a report of two cases. *Skeletal Radiol* 1987;16:316–319.

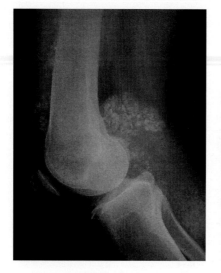

FIGURE 5.65A

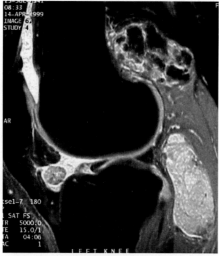

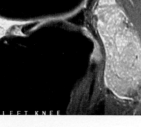

FIGURE 5.65C

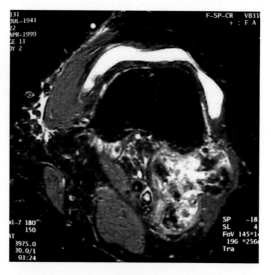

FIGURE 5.65B

FIGURE 5.65D

CLINICAL HISTORY

Knee pain and swelling.

FINDINGS

The lateral radiograph of the knee demonstrates multiple small rounded regions of soft-tissue ossification conforming to the outline of a distended knee joint. On the sagittal proton-density-weighted image, multiple lobulated masses with intermediate and high signal intensities are noted within the joint and around the femur (Fig. 5.65A). On the sagittal STIR (Fig. 5.65C) and axial fat-suppressed proton-density images (Fig. 5.65D), there is an effusion, as well as a heterogeneous mass with low, intermediate, and high signal within a distended superior recess of the knee joint. Several rounded regions of the mass show signal characteristics of fat, consistent with bone marrow (Fig. 5.65B–C).

DIAGNOSIS

Idiopathic synovial osteochondromatosis.

DISCUSSION

Idiopathic synovial osteochondromatosis is an uncommon benign disorder caused by metaplasia of the synovium and the intrasynovial formation of cartilaginous nodules. These nodules progressively become ossified and can separate from the synovium to lie loose within the affected articulation. Idiopathic synovial osteochondromatosis is always monoarticular and most commonly involves the knee (1,2). The disorder can be seen at all ages but most commonly affects young and middle-aged adults (3,4). Clinically, patients present with pain, swelling, and occasionally, locking or restricted knee motion (2).

In the early stages of the disorder, prior to the development of ossification within the nodules, conventional radiographs show only an effusion within the joint. Later, innumerable calcified and ossified nodules outlining the synovium of the articulation can be identified, often with associated nonadherent calcified or ossified intraarticular bodies. In a tight articulation, such as the hip, there are frequently well-defined pressure erosions of the periarticular bony cortex. In the knee, which is a capacious joint, osseous erosion is rare (4).

The MR imaging findings of idiopathic synovial osteochondromatosis are likewise dependent on the stage of the disease. When the intrasynovial cartilage nodules are not calcified or ossified, their signal intensity is similar to fluid, namely, low on T1-weighted and high on T2-weighted sequences. At the early stages, it is difficult to recognize the chondroid metaplasia of the cartilage on conventional MR sequences. When the intrasynovial cartilage starts to become calcified, small, rounded areas of low signal intensities are noted on both T1- and T2-weighted images. As the lobules of cartilage become progressively ossified, ringlike structures with peripheral rims of low signal intensity and central regions of higher signal intensity similar to fatty marrow can be identified (4).

REFERENCES

1. Crotty JM, Monu JU, Pope TL, Jr. Synovial osteochondromatosis. *Radiol Clin North Am* 1996;34:327–342.
2. Valmassy R, Ferguson H. Synovial osteochondromatosis. A brief review. *J Am Podiatr Med Assoc* 1992;82:427–431.
3. Maurice H, Crone M, Watt I. Synovial chondromatosis. *J Bone Joint Surg [Br]* 1988;70:807–811.
4. Resnick D, Niwayama G. Soft tissue. In: Resnick D, Niwayama G, eds. *Diagnosis of bone and joint disorders*, 3rd ed. Philadelphia: WB Saunders, 1996:Chapter 95.

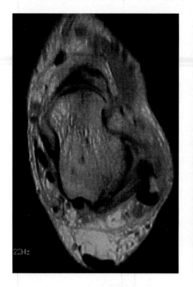

FIGURE 6.66A

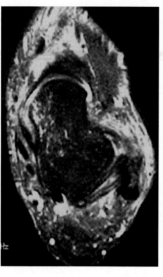

FIGURE 6.66B

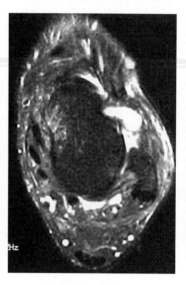

FIGURE 6.66C

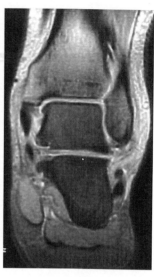

FIGURE 6.66D

CLINICAL HISTORY

This 44-year-old woman twisted her ankle.

FINDINGS

The axial T1-weighted image at the level of the midtalus (Fig. 6.66A) shows soft-tissue thickening around the distal fibula. The fibular attachment of the anterior talofibular ligament is disrupted. The posterior talofibular ligament is intact. Fat-suppressed T2-weighted axial images (Fig. 6.66B–C) of the same region confirm the rupture of the an-terior talofibular ligament at its fibular attachment site. Articular fluid extends through the gap into the adjacent soft tissues. Extensive soft-tissue edema is evident around the lateral ankle. The coronal fat-suppressed proton-density image (Fig. 6.66D) shows that the deltoid ligament and the calcane-ofibular ligament are intact.

DIAGNOSIS

Tear of the anterior talofibular ligament.

DISCUSSION

There are four major ligamentous complexes around the ankle that stabilize the ankle articulation. These four liga-mentous complexes are the lateral collateral ligament, the deltoid ligament, the syndesmotic complex, and the talo-calcaneal ligaments of the sinus tarsi (1,2). The lateral col-lateral ligament is composed of three major ligaments: the anterior talofibular, posterior talofibular, and calcaneofibu-lar ligaments. These ligaments stabilize the lateral aspect of the ankle joint. The medially located deltoid ligament is divided into superficial and deep layers. The syndesmotic complex includes the anterior tibiofibular, posterior tibiofibular, and interosseous ligaments. This group of lig-aments stabilizes the distal tibiofibular joint. The talo-calcaneal ligament is formed by a portion of the extensor retinaculum, the cervical ligament, and the talocalcaneal interosseous ligament.

Ankle ligament sprains are very common, accounting for thousands of doctor visits each day in the United States. The lateral collateral ligament complex is the most common site of soft-tissue injury about the ankle, comprising approximately 85% of all ligamentous injuries in this region (1,3). The mechanism of injury is most commonly a fall or a twisting injury with the foot planted. Most ankle injuries are caused by excessive inversion of the foot in plantar flexion, resulting in sequential tearing of the lateral collateral ligaments from anterior to posterior. The anterior talofibular ligament is torn first, followed by the calcaneofibular ligament, and finally, by the posterior talofibular ligament. Complete tears of the posterior calcaneofibular ligament are uncommon and are often associated with dislocation of the tibiotalar joint.

Injuries of the ligaments are referred to as sprains and are classified into three grades based on their severity. A grade 1 sprain is defined as stretching of the ligament producing microscopic tears within its substance. Clinically, mild swelling and tenderness are present, but the joint remains stable. A grade 2 sprain is a partial macroscopic tear of the ligament associated with moderate swelling and pain, as well as mild or moderate articular laxity. A grade 3 sprain represents a complete rupture of the ligament and produces severe swelling and pain overlying the injury. There is loss of function of the injured joint due to the profound laxity produced by a grade 3 ankle ligament injury (3,4).

MR imaging is not routinely obtained for evaluation of ligament injuries about the ankle. The MR examination can be valuable in the high-performance athlete to help plan ankle reconstruction or in the patient with an equivocal clinical examination (4). To evaluate the lateral ligaments on MR adequately, proper positioning of the foot is important. The anterior talofibular ligament is horizontally oriented, with a slightly descending course as it extends from the an-terior margin of the lateral malleolus to its talar attachment. The posterior talofibular ligament also has a horizontal course as it passes from lateral malleolus to posterior talus. Therefore the full length of the ligament can be seen on axial images when the foot is in the neutral or the dorsiflexed position (2,5). Both ligaments are best seen at the level of the distal fibular notch, which produces a prominent posteromedial concavity at the distal fibular tip. The calcaneofibular ligament has a relatively vertical course as it passes from the distal fibula posteroinferiorly toward its attachment on the lateral calcaneus. This ligament is best visualized on the coronal images that show the distal fibula.

Like all ligaments in the body, the lateral collateral ligaments of the ankle are normally homogeneous low signal intensity on both T1- and T2-weighted images. Injuries of the ligaments are easiest to identify when they are acute and there are overlying soft-tissue edema and intraarticular fluid. Chronic injuries are more difficult to visualize, as effusion is typically absent so the only MR findings are thickening or irregularity of the injured ligament. In the absence of an effusion, MR arthrography can improve the diagnostic accuracy of the examination (2,3). Mild ligament sprains produce thickening of the ligament and high signal within its fibers, as well as edema in the overlying soft tissues. When the ligament is torn, the ligament may appear lax and wavy. Disruption or attenuation of the ligament due to a macroscopic tear produces high signal in the region of the tear on T2-weighted images. Discontinuity or absence of the ligament can be identified, particularly if there is sufficient joint effusion to outline the gap produced by the ligamentous rupture. Effusion extravasates out of the joint capsule into the surrounding soft tissue, providing excellent contrast for identifying the torn ligaments.

REFERENCES

1. Horton MG, Timins ME. MR imaging of injuries to the small joints. *Radiol Clin North Am* 1997;35:671–700.
2. Mesgarzadeh M, Schneck CD, Tehranzadeh J, et al. Magnetic resonance imaging of ankle ligaments: emphasis on anatomy and injuries to lateral collateral ligaments. *Magn Reson Imaging Clin N Am* 1994;2:39–58.
3. Haygood TM. Magnetic resonance imaging of the musculoskeletal system: Part 7. The ankle. *Clin Orthop* 1997;Mar(336):318–336.
4. Frey C, Bell J, Teresi L, et al. A comparison of MRI and clinical examination of acute lateral ankle sprains. *Foot Ankle Int* 1996;17:533–537.
5. Resnick D, Kang HS. Ankle and foot. In: Resnick D, Kang HS, eds. *Internal derangements of joints.* Philadelphia: WB Saunders, 1997:823–838.

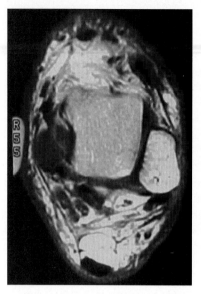 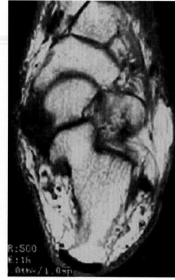 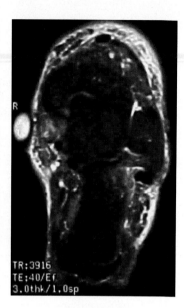

| FIGURE 6.67A | FIGURE 6.67B | FIGURE 6.67C |

CLINICAL HISTORY

A middle-aged woman complained of chronic foot pain.

FINDINGS

An axial T1-weighted image through the tibiotalar joint (Fig. 6.67A) and a more distal image at the level of the talonavicular joint (Fig. 6.67B) demonstrate enlargement of the posterior tibial tendon sheath. Intermediate signal intensity filled the tendon sheath from the level of the distal fibula to the base of the metatarsals. The coronal fat-suppressed proton-density-weighted image (Fig. 6.67C) shows increased signal intensity within the posterior tibial tendon sheath. The normal low signal intensity of the posterior tibial tendon is not visualized.

DIAGNOSIS

Complete rupture of the posterior tibial tendon.

DISCUSSION

The posterior tibialis muscle originates from the proximal third of the posterior tibia and the interosseous membrane. Its myotendinous junction lies within the distal third of the leg. The entire tendon is surrounded by a synovial tendon sheath. The posterior tibial tendon courses distally, curves behind the medial malleolus, and then passes anteriorly through the flexor retinaculum, superficial to the tibiotalar and tibiocalcaneal components of the deltoid ligament. Most of the tendon fibers insert onto the navicular tuberosity. The remaining fibers insert onto the plantar aspect of the cuboid, cuneiform, and middle three metatarsals (1,2). The primary function of the posterior tibialis is to invert and plantarflex the hindfoot. In addition, the posterior tibial tendon maintains the medial longitudinal arch of the foot and the mild valgus position of the hindfoot.

Up to 67% of cases of posterior tibial tendon dysfunction are seen in middle-aged or elderly women (1,3). More than 90% of cases are unilateral, with a slight left-sided predominance (1,3). Acute trauma to the tendon is uncommon, occurring predominantly in younger people. Posterior tibial tendon insufficiency is usually chronic in nature, caused by repetitive microtrauma and chronic microdegeneration of the tendon from altered mechanics of the foot. The tendon is also commonly damaged due to inflammatory disorders such as rheumatoid arthritis, seronegative spondyloarthropathies, systemic lupus erythematosus, and gout. Obesity, diabetes mellitus, hypertension, and local or systemic use of corticosteroids also increase the risk of posterior tibial tendon tear (1,3). Clinically, patients present with chronic medial foot pain that is worsened by weight bearing. Tenderness, edema, and warmth along the medial hindfoot may be present. An acquired flatfoot deformity with hindfoot valgus and forefoot abduction and pronation progressively develops. Patients have weakness in inverting the foot and are unable to raise their heel off the ground when standing only on the affected foot (4,5).

Tears of the posterior tibial tendon are most commonly located at the level of the medial malleolus, where the tendon makes a sharp turn to course anteriorly under the bony prominence. A considerable amount of frictional force is exerted on the tendon in this region. The hypovascularity of this region of the tendon is another factor that predisposes this region to a tear. From the initial site of tendon damage, tears can propagate proximally or distally (1,3). Another common site of tendon tear is adjacent to the attachment of the tendon on the navicular tuberosity. Tendinopathy, rupture, and avulsion of the posterior tibial tendon can all develop at this distal portion of the tendon.

MR imaging is an excellent modality for evaluating posterior tibial tendon tears, particularly in the early stages of the disease when clinical diagnosis is difficult. Early diagnosis is important as prompt treatment can prevent secondary foot deformity. The sensitivity and specificity of MR imaging for tears of the posterior tibial tendon have been reported as 95% and 100%, respectively (3). Images should be obtained with the foot in either neutral or a slightly plantar flexed position. The axial and sagittal images of the ankle are most useful for assessment of this structure. The posterior tibial tendon is the most medial tendon in the posterior compartment. It lies immediately behind the medial malleolus, just anterior to the flexor digitorum and flexor hallucis tendons. It is the largest of the tendons adjacent to the medial malleolus, with a normal diameter about two to three times larger than the flexor digitorum longus and flexor hallucis longus. The normal tendon appears homogeneous with low signal intensity on both T1- and T2-weighted sequences, except for its insertion site on the navicular, where the tendon is often slightly heterogeneous with intermediate signal. Normally, there is either no or only a scant amount of fluid is within the tendon sheath.

Tears of the posterior tibial tendon have been classified into three different patterns (1–3). The type I tear is a partial tear with microtears and longitudinal splits within the tendon, usually on its undersurface. The tendon is thickened due to edema, hemorrhage, and scarring, and appears considerably larger than its normal size. Foci of increased signal intensity are seen on T1- and proton-density-weighted images, but the tendon remains low signal on T2-weighted sequences. As the posterior tibial tendon progressively degenerates, a type II partial tear develops. In a type II tear, there is increased splitting, elongation, and stretching of the tendons, leading to an atretic appearance. The tendon becomes focally narrowed to an equal or smaller diameter than the adjacent flexor digitorum longus tendon. The tendon can be hypertrophied proximal and distal to the narrowed segment. A type III tear is a complete tear of the posterior tibial tendon. Discontinuity of the tendon or uniform degeneration of the tendon is noted. Signal abnormalities are evident on the T2-weighted sequences, which show the gap and retraction of the tendon to its greatest advantage. The tendon sheath is filled with fluid, fat, or mucinous degeneration. Extensive fluid within the tendon sheath suggests tenosynovitis, which is commonly associated with a partial tear of the tendon. Other abnormalities associated with the posterior tibial dysfunction are also noted, such as thickening of the flexor retinaculum and edema of the medial soft tissues.

REFERENCES

1. Khoury NJ, el-Khoury GY, Saltzman CL, et al. MR imaging of posterior tibial tendon dysfunction. *AJR* 1996;167:675–682.
2. Conti SF. Posterior tibial tendon problems in athletes. *Orthop Clin North Am* 1994;25:109–121.
3. Rosenberg ZS. Chronic rupture of the posterior tibial tendon. *Magn Reson Imaging Clin N Am* 1994;2:79–87.
4. Hogan JF. Posterior tibial tendon dysfunction and MRI. *J Foot Ankle Surg* 1993;32:467–472.
5. Lim PS, Schweitzer ME, Deely DM, et al. Posterior tibial tendon dysfunction: secondary MR signs. *Foot Ankle Int* 1997;18:658–663.

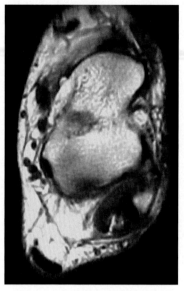

FIGURE 6.68A

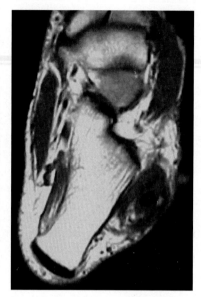

FIGURE 6.68B

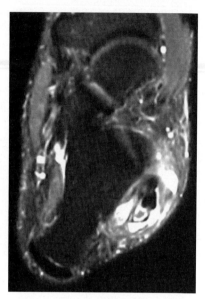

FIGURE 6.68C

CLINICAL HISTORY

A 52-year-old man with foot pain.

FINDINGS

The axial T1 images (Fig. 6.68A–B) of the ankle demonstrate abnormal intermediate signal intensity of the peroneus brevis tendon. The peroneus brevis tendon is not visualized, and there is fragmented low-signal material in its expected position anterior to the peroneus longus. Amorphous signal intensity is also noted in the sheath and soft tissues surrounding the peroneus longus and brevis tendons. On the fat-suppressed proton-density image (Fig. 6.68C), high-signal-intensity material surrounds the peroneus longus and brevis tendons. There is a large amount of fluid in the tendon sheath. High signal intensity is seen within the peroneus brevis tendon.

DIAGNOSIS

Tear of the peroneus brevis tendon.

DISCUSSION

The peroneus longus and peroneus brevis muscles occupy the lateral compartment of the leg. These muscles are lateral stabilizers of the ankle and foot, and function to elevate and evert the foot. The peroneus longus arises from the lateral condyle of the tibia, the intermuscular septum, and the proximal fibula. The peroneus brevis arises from the midfibula and the distal fibula. The peroneus brevis muscle normally lies deep to the peroneus longus above the ankle (1–3). At the level of the ankle, these two tendons come together behind the lateral malleolus and are surrounded by a common synovial sheath that curves below the fibula to pass lateral to the calcaneus. This common sheath separates into two sheaths at the level of the calcaneocuboid joint.

Two fascial thickenings, the superior and inferior peroneal retinaculae, hold the peroneal tendons within the retromalleolar groove behind the lateral malleolus. At this level, as the two tendons turn anteriorly around the distal lateral malleolus, the peroneus brevis lies anterior to the peroneus longus. Lateral to the calcaneus, the tendons are separated by the peroneal tubercle of the calcaneus. The peroneus brevis tendon inserts on the base of the fifth metatarsal, and the peroneus longus tendon inserts on the first metatarsal and medial cuneiform.

Abnormalities of the peroneal tendons include tendinopathy, tenosynovitis, tendinitis, tears, and subluxations (1,2,4,5). Tendinopathy is a degenerative phenomenon that is uncommon in the peroneal compartment. Tenosynovitis and tendinitis of the tendons have various causes, including acute trauma, chronic stress, abnormal foot mechanics caused by conditions such as tarsal coalition, inflammatory arthritides, congenital or acquired hypertrophy of the peroneal tubercle, and idiopathic etiologies. In both tendinitis and tenosynovitis, MR imaging shows significant amounts of fluid surrounding the peroneal tendons within their tendon sheath. If tendinitis is present, the tendon often appears thickened and irregular. Increased signal intensity on T1- and proton-density-weighted images is seen within the tendon, which normally appears homogeneously dark on T1-weighted images. When a large amount of fluid is present within the sheath, attention should be directed to the calcaneofibular ligament. Tears of the calcaneofibular ligament allow communication of the ankle joint with the peroneal tendon sheath, allowing joint fluid to extend into the sheath, simulating tenosynovitis.

Peroneal tendons can be partially torn or completely ruptured. Tears are commonly due to acute injury, but they may occur spontaneously in a degenerated tendon. Acute rupture usually occurs in young athletes who acutely injure the ankle with forcible contraction of the peroneus. Peroneal tendon tears typically start near the tip of the lateral malleolus, where the stress is maximal. From this point the tears propagate distally or proximally. The most common type of tear is a longitudinal split of the peroneus brevis tendon (2,5). Longitudinal tears of the peroneus brevis are much more common than tears involving the peroneus longus. This type of tear represents 11% to 37% of all peroneal tendon injuries (1). When the longitudinal split is extensive, the peroneus brevis tendon divides into two parts and surrounds the peroneus longus. These tears produce a linear band of high signal within the substance of the tendon on T2-weighted images. On the axial images, the peroneus brevis tendon appears to be C-shaped or like a boomerang in appearance as it wraps around the peroneus longus tendon. Concomitant tears of the peroneus longus tendon at the level of the lateral malleolus have been noted in 16% to 29% of the cases.

Isolated acute tears of the peroneus longus typically occur at the level of the calcaneocuboid joint, distal to the os peroneum or less commonly at the level of this sesamoid bone. Complete tears of the peroneal tendons are well seen on both axial and sagittal MR images. The MR images show disruption or absence of the normal dark-signal-intensity tendon, with no continuity of tendon fibers. Fluid or hemorrhage fills the gap, giving amorphous signal intensity on T1- or proton-density-weighted images and high signal intensity on T2-weighted images.

Subluxation and dislocation of the peroneal tendons are uncommon. Peroneal subluxation is most commonly due to traumatic insufficiency of the superior retinaculum or a congenitally shallow retromalleolar groove (1,2,4). The tendons usually subluxate or dislocate anterolaterally out of the retromalleolar groove, around the lateral malleolus, to lie lateral to the lateral malleolus. Recurrent subluxation of the tendons may lead to peroneus brevis tendon split syndrome. MR can be utilized to evaluate the position and integrity of the tendons in patients with recurrent subluxation. Not only can MR detect the dislocation, anatomic variation of the ankle bony structure and the integrity of the tendons can also be evaluated. Positioning the foot in eversion may be necessary to allow recognition of positional subluxation of the peroneal tendons.

REFERENCES

1. Mota J, Rosenberg ZS. Magnetic resonance imaging of the peroneal tendons. *Top Magn Reson Imaging* 1998;9:273–285.
2. Ton ER, Schweitzer ME, Karasick D. MR imaging of peroneal tendon disorders. *AJR* 1997;168:135–140.
3. Sammarco GJ. Peroneal tendon injuries. *Orthop Clin North Am* 1994;25:135–145.
4. Chandnani VP, Bradley YC. Achilles tendon and miscellaneous tendon lesions. *Magn Reson Imaging Clin N Am* 1994;2:89–96.
5. Khoury NJ, el-Khoury GY, Saltzman CL, et al. Peroneus longus and brevis tendon tears: MR imaging evaluation. *Radiology* 1996;200:833–841.

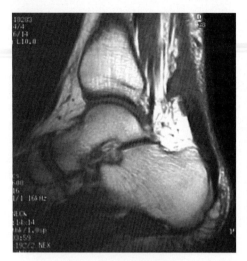

FIGURE 6.69A

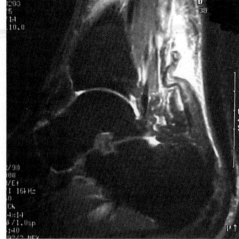

FIGURE 6.69B

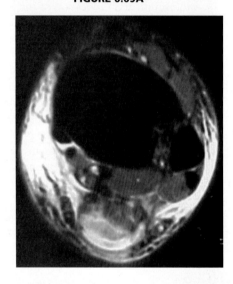

FIGURE 6.69C

CLINICAL HISTORY

A 38-year-old man injured his ankle and was unable to walk.

FINDINGS

The sagittal T1-weighted image (Fig. 6.69A) demonstrates disruption of the Achilles tendon at its musculotendinous junction. The normal low-signal tendon is replaced by irregular tissue of intermediate signal intensity. The sagittal short tau inversion recover (STIR) image (Fig. 6.69B) also shows disruption of the Achilles tendon a few centimeters proximal to its calcaneal attachment site and high signal within the substance of the tendon. The tendon is wavy and thickened. On the fat-suppressed proton-density image (Fig. 6.69C), the tendon has lost its normal oval shape and anterior concavity. Soft-tissue edema is present around the tendon and in the pre-Achilles fat pad.

DIAGNOSIS

Rupture of the Achilles tendon.

DISCUSSION

The Achilles tendon is formed by the tendons of the gastrocnemius and soleus muscles. The medial and lateral heads of the gastrocnemius arise from the medial and lateral femoral condyles, respectively. The two heads merge together and are joined distally by the soleus, which arises from the proximal tibia and fibula and lies deep to the gastrocnemius muscle in the leg (1,2). The Achilles tendon is the largest tendon in the body. It extends approximately 8 cm distally from its myotendinous junction to insert onto the superior calcaneal tuberosity. The proximal tendon is rounded, whereas the distal tendon is relatively flattened in the sagittal plane, with a mild anterior concavity and a convex posterior margin. The fibers of the Achilles tendon spiral 90 degrees so that the soleal portion of the tendon inserts medial to the gastrocnemius portion of the tendon on the calcaneus. This configuration allows improved tendon elongation and elastic recoil. The Achilles tendon is surrounded by a paratenon rather than a synovial sheath (1). Abnormalities of the Achilles tendon include myxoid degeneration (tendinopathy), inflammation of the tendon (tendinitis), partial tear, and rupture of the tendon. Inflammation can also develop in the paratenon around the tendon, leading to paratendinitis or peritendinitis (3).

The mechanism of Achilles tendon abnormalities appears to be multifactorial. Proposed etiologies for tendon damage include biomechanical injuries, inflammatory and autoimmune conditions, genetic collagen abnormalities, drugs, infectious disorders, and neurologic conditions (1,2,4,5). Tendinopathy and tears are especially common in athletes, particularly among runners and those involved in jumping activities associated with forced dorsiflexion of the foot. Tears can also be seen in sedentary people who participate in occasional strenuous exercise. Overuse or misuse of the foot and ankle causes microtears and inflammation of the tendon and the area around the tendon, particularly in the region about 3 cm proximal to the insertion, where the blood supply is relatively diminished. Common inflammatory conditions that lead to peritendinitis or tendinitis and subsequent rupture of the tendon include rheumatoid arthritis, systemic lupus erythematosus, primary and secondary hyperparathyroidism, and rarely, gout. Anabolic hormones and corticosteroids cause dysplasia of the tendon fibers, which predisposes to tear or rupture of the tendon.

Abnormalities of the Achilles tendon are more common in men than in women. The peak age is the third through fifth decades. Clinically, patients present with pain and swelling. Patients experience severe pain as they try to stand on the toes of the affected leg. In complete rupture, the patient is unable to stand on the toes and a palpable gap in the tendon may be detected.

The most common abnormality seen involving the Achilles tendon is degenerative tendinopathy. Tendinopathy produces thickening of the tendon, which assumes a more rounded shape, with loss of the normal anterior concavity of the distal portion of the tendon. The tendon remains low signal on T1- and T2-weighted sequences. If peritendinitis or paratendinitis is present, the T2-weighted images show increased signal intensity around the tendon and in the pre-Achilles fat. When high signal intensity is observed within the tendon on the T2-weighted sequences, a partial or complete tear of the tendon is likely present (3). Partial or complete tears of the tendon show disruption of the Achilles tendon fibers. In a partial tear, some of the fibers maintain continuity and there is only an incomplete gap in the tendon. Partial tears can be longitudinal or transverse. The axial images are best for detection of residual intact fibers in this type of tear. In the presence of a complete tear, the torn tendon may be retracted proximally and distally, leaving a gap that fills with high-signal-intensity hemorrhage and edema. The underlying tendon is often abnormal, showing changes of preexisting tendinopathy. MR imaging is also useful for assessment of the postoperative tendon, as recurrent ruptures of the tendon are seen in 10% of the conservatively managed group and 4% of the surgically treated group (5).

REFERENCES

1. Scioli MW. Achilles tendinitis. *Orthop Clin North Am* 1994;25:177–182.
2. Myerson MS, McGarvey W. Disorders of the Achilles tendon insertion and Achilles tendinitis. *Instr Course Lect* 1999;48:211–218.
3. Chandnani VP, Bradley YC. Achilles tendon and miscellaneous tendon lesions. *Magn Reson Imaging Clin N Am* 1994;2:89–96.
4. Leppilahti J, Orava S. Total Achilles tendon rupture. A review. *Sports Med* 1998;25:79–100.
5. Maffulli N. Rupture of the Achilles tendon. *J Bone Joint Surg [Am]* 1999;81:1019–1036.

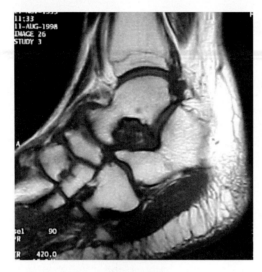

FIGURE 6.70A

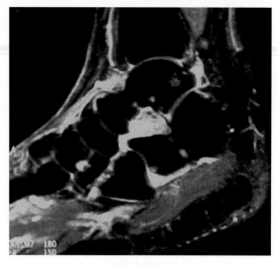

FIGURE 6.70B

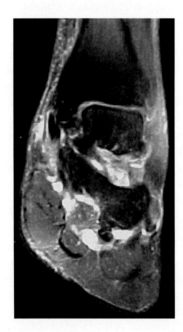

FIGURE 6.70C

CLINICAL HISTORY

A 62-year-old woman with lateral ankle pain.

FINDINGS

The sagittal T1-weighted image (Fig. 6.70A) demonstrates diffuse low signal intensity replacing the fat within the sinus tarsi. On the sagittal STIR image (Fig. 6.70B) and coronal fat-suppressed proton-density-weighted image (Fig. 6.70C), the entire sinus tarsi contains tissue of increased signal intensity. The interosseous ligament and the cervical ligament are not visualized. Small cystic lesions are noted in the talus and calcaneus adjacent to the sinus tarsi and posterior subtalar joint.

DIAGNOSIS

Sinus tarsi syndrome.

DISCUSSION

The sinus tarsi is a cone-shaped space between the posterior subtalar joint and the anterior talocalcaneonavicular joint. The space is inferior to the midportion of the talus and superior to the calcaneus. The opening of the cone is located anterolaterally, representing the tarsal sinus proper. As the cone extends posteromedially, it narrows with its apex located just behind the sustentaculum tali. This narrow portion is termed the *tarsal canal* (1–3). The normal sinus tarsi contains fat, an arterial anastomosis between the posterior tibial and peroneal arteries, nerve endings, synovium, and capsular from the adjacent articulations, as well as five ligaments. These five ligaments are the medial, intermediate, and lateral roots of the inferior extensor retinaculum laterally, the cervical ligament in the anterior tarsal sinus, and the interosseous talocalcaneal ligament (the ligament of the tarsal canal) posteromedially (1). The ligaments maintain alignment between the talus and calcaneus and limit inversion of the foot.

Injury to the structures in the sinus tarsi produces sinus tarsi syndrome, which consists of chronic lateral foot pain, focal tenderness to palpation, and the subjective perception of hindfoot instability (1,4). Seventy percent of cases of sinus tarsi syndrome are caused by inversion injury to the ankle. Other causes of sinus tarsi syndrome include inflammatory disorders such as ankylosing spondylitis, rheumatoid arthritis and gout, and foot deformities such as pes cavus or pes planus. As most cases are due to inversion trauma, there is a high association with tears of the lateral collateral ligaments of the ankle (1,3). Seventy-nine percent of patients who have an abnormal sinus tarsi also have tears of the lateral collateral ligaments, whereas 39% of patients with lateral collateral ligament injury have abnormalities of the tarsal sinus and canal (2). Although patients often complain of a sensation that the hindfoot is unstable, radiographs and clinical examinations usually do not provide objective evidence of subtalar joint instability. Lateral foot pain is most severe while standing or walking, or with supination and abduction of the foot. The pain typically resolves with rest. Local anesthetic injection in the area of the sinus tarsi reduces the pain and sensation of instability.

There are no specific radiographic findings in sinus tarsi syndrome. Contrast injection into the posterior subtalar joint can show obliteration of the normal synovial recesses about the talocalcaneal interosseous ligament and leakage of contrast material into the sinus tarsi. Although these arthrographic findings are suggestive of sinus tarsi syndrome, this technique is not sensitive (1,2,4).

MR imaging has been employed to diagnose sinus tarsi syndrome and has shown high accuracy for evaluation of the sinus tarsi. All three imaging planes are important for visualization of the contents of this region (3,4). Normally, the sinus tarsi contains predominantly fatty tissue, interspersed with oblique linear low-signal bands representing the inferior extensor retinaculum, the cervical ligament, and the interosseous ligament as one progresses from lateral to medial. In sinus tarsi syndrome, the normal fat is replaced by inflammatory tissue and hypertrophied synovium, producing low signal intensity on T1- and high signal intensity on T2-weighted sequences. Abnormal fluid collections within the sinus tarsi can also be present. In severe cases, small fluid collections extend into the adjacent soft tissues from the region of the sinus tarsi. The cervical ligament and the interosseous ligament are often not seen or poorly defined. Subchondral cysts at the insertion of the ligaments are occasionally formed (1). In chronic cases, diffuse low signal intensity can be seen on both sequences due to fibrosis within the tarsal sinus. Advanced disease leads to secondary osteoarthritis of the posterior subtalar joint, with cysts and bone marrow edema of the talus or calcaneus about the ligamentous insertions (1,3).

The ligaments and tendons about the ankle should be carefully evaluated if abnormalities are present in the tarsal sinus due to the high association of other soft-tissue injuries with this syndrome. The most frequently torn ligaments are the anterior talofibular and the calcaneofibular ligaments on the lateral side of the ankle. The most characteristic ligament injury associated with sinus tarsi syndrome is a tear of the calcaneofibular ligament (3). Tears of the tibialis posterior tendon are also frequently associated with sinus tarsi syndrome.

REFERENCES

1. Steinbach LS. Painful syndromes around the ankle and foot: magnetic resonance imaging evaluation. *Top Magn Reson Imaging* 1998;9:311–326.
2. Klein MA, Spreitzer AM. MR imaging of the tarsal sinus and canal: normal anatomy, pathologic findings, and features of the sinus tarsi syndrome. *Radiology* 1993;186:233–240.
3. Beltran J. Sinus tarsi syndrome. *Magn Reson Imaging Clin N Am* 1994;2:59–65.
4. Resnick D, Kang HS. Ankle and foot. In: Resnick D, Kang HS, eds. *Internal derangements of joints.* Philadelphia: WB Saunders, 1997:823–839.

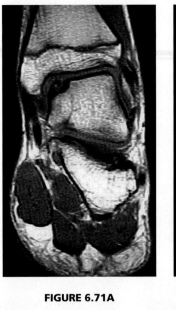

FIGURE 6.71A

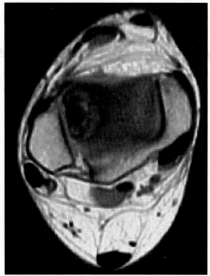

FIGURE 6.71B

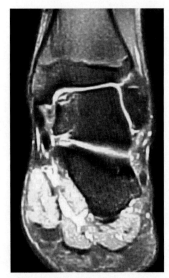

FIGURE 6.71C

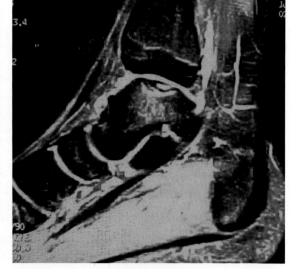

FIGURE 6.71D

CLINICAL HISTORY

A 15-year-old boy complained of ankle discomfort.

FINDINGS

The coronal T1-weighted image (Fig. 6.71A) shows a crescentic region of low signal in the subchondral region of the medial talar dome. On the axial T1-weighted sequence (Fig. 6.71B), the medial articular surface of the talus has irregular decreased signal and appears fragmented. Curvilinear high signal is present at the base of this lesion on the coronal (Fig. 6.71C) and sagittal (Fig. 6.71D) fat-suppressed proton-density-weighted images. The sagittal image also demonstrates considerable marrow edema surrounding the bony defect. The overlying cortex is discontinuous and flattened. There is a small effusion within the joint. No intraarticular bodies are identified.

DIAGNOSIS

Osteochondritis dissecans of the medial talar dome.

DISCUSSION

Osteochondritis dissecans (OCD) of the talus represents fragmentation, and potential separation, of a portion of the subchondral bone, and sometimes the overlying articular cartilage. Clinical presentation is usually during adolescence, with males affected more frequently than females [1]. OCD of the talus is less common than OCD in the knee or elbow [1]. The etiology of OCD of the talus is unclear but is thought to be a chronic osteochondral injury resulting from transmission of tangential shearing forces across the joint space. Abnormal alignment or ligamentous laxity predisposes the ankle to excessive shearing forces. Other proposed etiologies include familial or hereditary cartilage abnormalities and microembolic events leading to avascular necrosis of the subchondral bone [1–3].

The lesions typically involve the medial or lateral corners of the talar dome [1,4]. Lateral lesions are located at the anterior talar corner and are thought to be due to inversion and dorsiflexion with fibular impingement on the talus. The lateral lesion appears thin and shallow with a waferlike appearance. OCD of the medial talar dome is more common. The medial lesion is more posteriorly located and is thought to be due to talar impaction during eversion and planter flexion of the foot. The medial lesion is typically larger, is more cup-shaped, and extends more deeply into the body of the talus.

Lesions of OCD are staged in a similar fashion regardless of their location in the body [4]. The stage I lesion of OCD is a subchondral fracture with intact overlying cartilage. The stage II lesion has a partially detached osteochondral fragment. Stage III lesions, like the one illustrated, consist of a completely detached fragment from the talus but the fragment is undisplaced. In a stage IV lesion, there is detachment of the osteochondral fragment from the underlying bone with displacement of the loose fragment [4].

MR is very accurate for diagnosing and staging of OCD. The morphology of the lesion, its interface with the native bone, and the status of the overlying cartilage can be assessed. Coronal and sagittal images are most useful for evaluating OCD of the talar dome. The lesion itself can be recognized by the presence of abnormal low signal within the marrow of the talar dome. The signal within the lesion is variable, depending partly on the viability of the fragment. Necrotic fragments typically demonstrate a larger size and lower internal signal than stable viable lesions [5]. The interface between the OCD and the talus appears low signal on T1-weighted sequences. The presence of high signal intensity between the lesion and the parent bone on T2-weighted sequences suggests granulation tissue or fluid at the interface and is considered a sign of instability of the lesion. The absence of such high signal generally indicates a stable lesion [5]. Focal defects in the cartilage and subchondral bone are another sign of instability. Such defects are produced by fragmentation and displacement of the unstable fragment from the parent bone. Assessment of the cartilage is problematic in the absence of a joint effusion. MR arthrography can be employed in this situation.

REFERENCES

1. Schoenberg NY, Lehman WB. Magnetic resonance imaging of pediatric disorders of the ankle and foot. *Magn Reson Imaging Clin N Am* 1994;2:109–122.
2. Clanton TO, DeLee JC. Osteochondritis dissecans: history, pathophysiology and current treatment concepts. *Clin Orthop* 1982;167:50–64.
3. Langer F, Percy EC. Osteochondritis dissecans and anomalous centres of ossification: a review of 80 lesions in 61 patients. *Can J Surg* 1971;14:208–215.
4. Horton MG, Timins ME. MR imaging of injuries to the small joints. *Radiol Clin North Am* 1997;35:671–700.
5. De Smet AA, Ilahi OA, Graf BK. Reassessment of the MR criteria for stability of osteochondritis dissecans in the knee and ankle. *Skeletal Radiol* 1996;25:159–163.

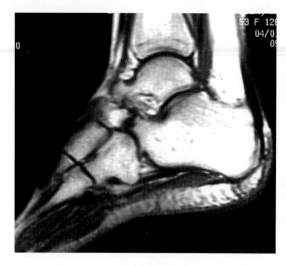 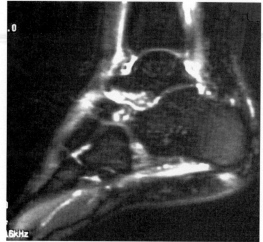

FIGURE 6.72A   **FIGURE 6.72B**

CLINICAL HISTORY

A middle-aged woman with foot pain and pes planus.

FINDINGS

The sagittal T1-weighted image (Fig. 6.72A) demonstrates a prominent anterosuperior process of the calcaneus. This enlarged calcaneal process abuts the navicular, with irregular low signal intensity between the two bones. On the corresponding sagittal STIR image (Fig. 6.72B), this junctional area is surrounded by bone marrow edema.

DIAGNOSIS

Calcaneonavicular coalition.

DISCUSSION

Tarsal coalition refers to fusion of two or more of the tarsal bones. It is a common condition, with an incidence of 1% to 2% in the general population. Although the exact cause of tarsal coalition is not known, it is thought that the condition is due to congenital or developmental failure of differentiation and segmentation of the developing mesenchyme (1–3). Cases are typically sporadic, though the condition does appear to run in families.

The most common location of tarsal coalition is between the talus and the calcaneus, followed by coalition between the calcaneus and the navicular. These two types of coalition comprise about 90% of the tarsal coalitions. Uncommon types of coalition include talonavicular and calcaneocuboid coalitions. The fusion of two tarsal bones may be fibrous tissue, cartilage, or bone. About half of patients have bilateral coalition. Bilaterality is most common with the calcaneonavicular type (1,4). Acquired coalition due to infection, trauma, articular disorders, or surgery does occur but is much less common than the developmental form of bone fusion (5).

The clinical presentation of tarsal coalition varies. Many cases are asymptomatic and detected as an incidental finding. The most common presenting symptom is pain (2,4,6,7). The typical onset of pain is during the second or third decades of life, though symptoms can present later. It is thought that symptoms develop when the fusion converts from a mobile fibrous or cartilaginous form to an ossified fusion as the patient ages. The onset of the pain may be insidious or associated with trauma. Restricted foot motion, cavus deformity, or peroneal spastic flat foot deformity may also be present (5). The symptoms of calcaneonavicular coalition are usually less severe than those of coalition of the other tarsal bones.

Coalition can be readily identified on conventional radiographs. In calcaneonavicular coalition, hypertrophy of the anterior process of the calcaneus, termed the *anteater nose sign,* can be seen on both the oblique and lateral foot views. The abnormal articulation between the anterior calcaneus and the navicular is best seen on a 45-degree oblique view of the foot (2,4,6). Subchondral sclerosis, osseous irregularity of the opposing bony surfaces, or a frank bony bar can be seen. Secondary signs include hypoplasia of the head of the talus, prominence of the anterosuperior talus, and talar beaking. In the presence of a continuous bony bar, MR imaging shows continuity of the cortex and marrow space between the fused bones. MR can also detect fibrous and cartilaginous coalitions, which can be overlooked on conventional radiographs. The coalition itself is low signal in these forms of fusion, but the reactive edema and cystic changes in the adjacent bone are well shown on MR imaging.

REFERENCES

1. Pachuda NM, Lasday SD, Jay RM. Tarsal coalition: etiology, diagnosis, and treatment. *J Foot Surg* 1990;29:474–488.
2. Cowell HR, Elener V. Rigid painful flatfoot secondary to tarsal coalition. *Clin Orthop* 1983;Jul-Aug(177):54–60.
3. Wheeler R, Guevera A, Bleck EE. Tarsal coalitions: review of the literature and case report of bilateral dual calcaneonavicular and talocalcaneal coalitions. *Clin Orthop* 1981;156:175–177.
4. Perlman MD, Wertheimer SJ. Tarsal coalitions. *J Foot Surg* 1986;25:58–67.
5. Resnick D, Kang HS. Ankle and foot. In: Resnick D, Kang HS, eds. *Internal derangements of joints.* Philadelphia: WB Saunders, 1997:877–879.
6. Percy EC, Mann DL. Tarsal coalition: a review of the literature and presentation of 13 cases. *Foot Ankle* 1988;9:40–44.
7. Stormont DM, Peterson HA. The relative incidence of tarsal coalition. *Clin Orthop* 1983;181:28–36.

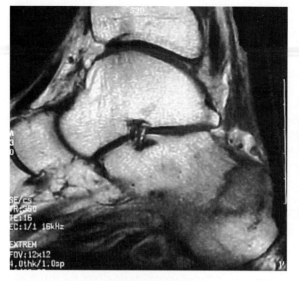

FIGURE 6.73A

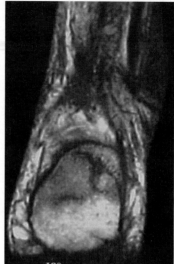

FIGURE 6.73B

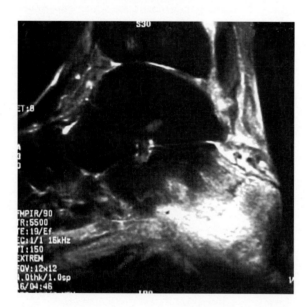

FIGURE 6.73C

CLINICAL HISTORY

A 64-year-old man complained of persistent atraumatic heel pain.

FINDINGS

The sagittal (Fig. 6.73A) and coronal (Fig. 6.73B) T1-weighted images of the hindfoot show irregular bands of low signal intensity in the calcaneal tuberosity. The bands of low signal are intramedullary and predominantly oriented perpendicular to the weight-bearing trabeculae. The lines extend to the cortical surface, but they do not involve the articular surface. On the sagittal STIR image (Fig. 6.73C), extensive edema is noted within the bone marrow of the calcaneus, as well as in the pre-Achilles fat pad and the plantar soft tissues. Persistent lines of low signal intensity are seen surrounded by high-signal bone marrow edema (Fig. 6.73C).

DIAGNOSIS

Insufficiency fracture of the calcaneus.

DISCUSSION

The calcaneus is the most common site of tarsal fracture, accounting for 60% of all tarsal fractures and 2% of all fractures in the body (1,2). Calcaneal fractures are generally classified into intraarticular and extraarticular types. Intraarticular fractures commonly occur as the result of a fall from a height, landing on the feet. The axial loading from such an injury drives the talus into the calcaneus. This type of fracture is often bilateral and has a poor prognosis due to articular surface incongruity leading to secondary osteoarthritis. Traumatic extraarticular fractures of the calcaneus are less common, accounting for 25% of all calcaneal fractures (2). Acute fractures of the calcaneus in children are rare, but when they do occur, most are extraarticular (1,2).

Nontraumatic stress fractures of the calcaneus are common and can be of the fatigue or insufficiency type. Stress fractures of the calcaneus account for up to 30% of stress fractures in military recruits and up to 15% of stress fractures in athletes (3). Fractures at this site can also be seen in patients with rheumatoid arthritis, neurologic disorders, and diseases leading to osteopenia. Typically, stress fractures are extraarticular and located in the posterior tuberosity of the calcaneus. Patients present with progressive heel pain without acute traumatic event. Radiographs are normal initially. Several weeks later, a vertical sclerotic band may develop, running from the posterosuperior surface into the cancellous part of the calcaneus, parallel to the posterior margin of the calcaneus. The sclerosis is perpendicular to the trabecular pattern of the bone.

Radionuclide bone scans and MR imaging are more sensitive than radiography for the early detection of a stress fracture. Early detection and treatment of stress fractures can dramatically decrease the morbidity. On MR examination, stress fractures of the calcaneus appear as low-signal-intensity lines in the intramedullary portion of the tuberosity, typically extending toward the superior cortex (3). Surrounding the low-signal-intensity lines are diffuse marrow edema and hemorrhage that appear as decreased signal intensity on T1- and increased signal intensity on T2-weighted images. The edema is most prominent within 3 weeks of the onset of symptoms. Edema can also be present in the adjacent soft tissue.

REFERENCES

1. Resnick D, Kang HS. Ankle and foot. In: Resnick D, Kang HS, eds. *Internal derangements of joints.* Philadelphia: WB Saunders 1997:813–815.
2. Kumar R, Matasar K, Stansberry S, et al. The calcaneus: normal and abnormal. *Radiographics* 1991;11:415–440.
3. Kier R. Magnetic resonance imaging of plantar fasciitis and other causes of heel pain. *Magn Reson Imaging Clin N Am* 1994;2:97–107.

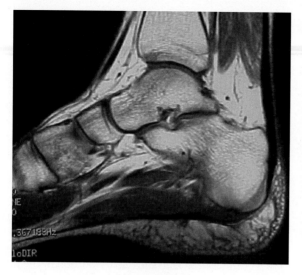

FIGURE 6.74A

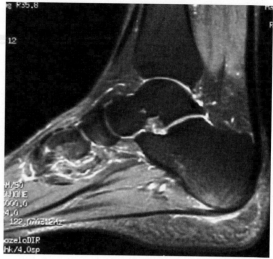

FIGURE 6.74B

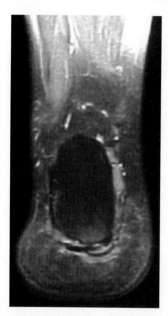

FIGURE 6.74C

CLINICAL HISTORY

A 35-year-old woman with heel pain.

FINDINGS

A sagittal T1-weighted image (Fig. 6.74A) at the level of the midportion of the calcaneus shows ill-defined low-signal-intensity streaky densities in the soft tissues adjacent to the plantar fascia. Sagittal (Fig. 6.74B) and coronal (Fig. 6.74C) fat-suppressed proton-density-weighted images show increased signal intensity in the deep and superficial soft tissues adjacent to the attachment of the plantar fascia to the calcaneus. Marrow edema is present in the calcaneus at the site of fascial attachment. The plantar fascia is slightly thickened (Fig. 6.74B).

DIAGNOSIS

Plantar fasciitis.

DISCUSSION

The plantar fascia, also known as the plantar aponeurosis, is a thick band of fibrous tissue on the plantar surface of the foot. It functions as an important static supporting structure for the longitudinal arch of the foot, acting as a bowstring on the plantar surface of the foot. The plantar fascia consists of multiple layers of fibrous tissue, which are divided into medial, central, and lateral bands. The central band of the plantar fascia is the thickest and strongest of these bands. The central band has a narrow origin at the posteromedial calcaneal tuberosity, just superficial to the flexor digitorum brevis muscle (1,2). As it extends distally, the plantar aponeurosis fans out into the skin and the proximal phalanges. The thinner and smaller medial and lateral portions are the fascial covering of the abductor hallucis and the abductor digiti minimi.

Plantar fasciitis represents inflammation of the plantar fascia and the perifascial tissues. It is regarded as the most common cause of inferior heel pain. Morning pain and stiffness, which improves after walking a few steps and is exacerbated by toe dorsiflexion, is the typical complaint (2–4). The onset of the pain is gradual with progressive worsening if the condition remains untreated. Treatment is typically conservative, consisting of rest, supportive shoes, and nonsteroidal antiinflammatory medication. Occasionally, local injection of a corticosteroid is necessary for adequate pain relief. Ten percent of patients are refractory to conservative management (3,4). Such patients benefit from partial surgical release of the medial fascia and decompression of the nerve supplying the abductor digiti quinti (3,4).

The etiologies of plantar fasciitis are divided into mechanical, degenerative, and systemic causes (5). Mechanical causes include overuse syndromes as well as conditions leading to malalignment of the foot. Disorders that alter the biomechanical forces transmitted through the foot, such as pes cavus, excessive pronation, and external rotation of the lower extremity, can all lead to inflammation of the plantar aponeurosis. Overuse can also lead to inflammation of the plantar fascia, especially among athletes such as runners, tennis players, basketball players, and dancers. Degenerative causes include atrophy of the heel pad and excessive foot pronation related to aging. Systemic causes include rheumatoid arthritis and other inflammatory arthritides.

MR imaging is an excellent tool for evaluating patients with persistent heel pain. Persistent heel pain can be caused by numerous conditions other than plantar fasciitis, including disorders such as calcaneal enthesophyte (heel spur), stress fracture of the calcaneus, Achilles tendinitis, pre-Achilles bursitis, and sinus tarsi syndrome. MR imaging can accurately identify the cause of heel pain among these myriad conditions. On MR examination, the normal plantar fascia appears as a homogeneous low-signal band on all sequences. It is normally only 2 to 4 mm thick along its entire course, with well-defined upper and lower margins. The fascia is surrounded by fatty tissue at its attachment on the calcaneus. When plantar fasciitis is present, the most common finding is perifascial edema, which causes ill-defined increased signal intensity in the perifascial fat on T2-weighted and STIR images. Superficial soft-tissue edema is more common and more prominent than edema in the tissues deep to the aponeurosis. Increased signal intensity may be seen within the plantar fascia on T2-weighted or STIR images owing to inflammation and microtears within the fascia (1,6,7). The fascia may be thickened, particularly at its calcaneal attachment site. Calcaneal marrow edema adjacent to the plantar fascia origin is occasionally present, giving rise to high signal intensity within the calcaneus on T2-weighted sequences.

REFERENCES

1. Steinbach LS. Painful syndromes around the ankle and foot: magnetic resonance imaging evaluation. *Top Magn Reson Imaging* 1998;9:311–326.
2. Schepsis AA, Leach RE, Gorzyca J. Plantar fasciitis: etiology, treatment, surgical results, and review of the literature. *Clin Orthop* 1991;May(266):185–196.
3. Tisdel CL, Donley BG, Sferra JJ. Diagnosing and treating plantar fasciitis: a conservative approach to plantar heel pain. *Cleve Clin J Med* 1999;66:231–235.
4. Barrett SJ, O'Malley R. Plantar fasciitis and other causes of heel pain. *Am Fam Physician* 1999;59:2200–2206.
5. Resnick D, Kang HS. Ankle and foot. In: Resnick D, Kang HS, eds. *Internal derangements of joints.* Philadelphia: WB Saunders, 1997:891–894.
6. Grasel RP, Schweitzer ME, Kovalovich AM, et al. MR imaging of plantar fasciitis: edema, tears, and occult marrow abnormalities correlated with outcome. *AJR* 1999;173:699–701.
7. Kier R, McCarthy S, Dietz MJ, et al. MR appearance of painful conditions of the ankle. *Radiographics* 1991;11:401–414.

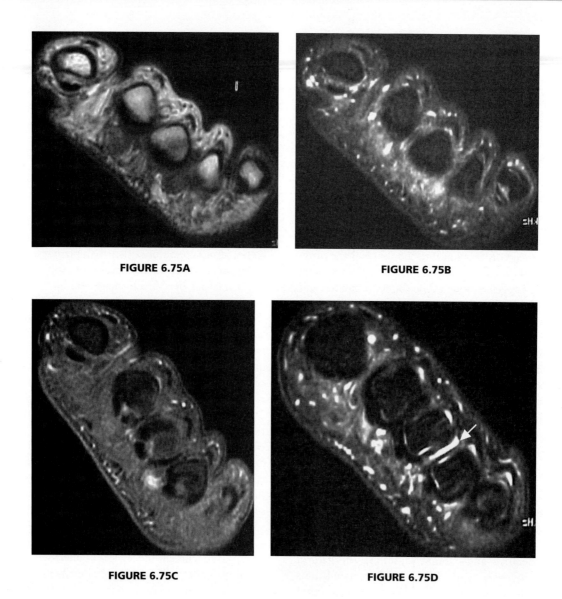

FIGURE 6.75A

FIGURE 6.75B

FIGURE 6.75C

FIGURE 6.75D

CLINICAL HISTORY

A 36-year-old woman complained of pain in the plantar tissues of her forefoot.

FINDINGS

An oblique coronal T1-weighted image of the forefoot shows an intermediate-signal-intensity mass located in the inferior interdigital space between the third and fourth metatarsophalangeal joints (Fig. 6.75A). On the oblique coronal fat-suppressed proton-density-weighted sequence (Fig. 6.75B), the mass has increased in signal intensity. The fat-suppressed T1-weighted image shows that the mass enhances brightly following the administration of intravenous gadolinium agent (Fig. 6.75C). Proximal to the mass, an elongated fluid collection is seen between the third and fourth metatarsal heads (Fig. 6.75D, *arrow*) on the T2-weighted image.

DIAGNOSIS

Morton's neuroma with associated intermetatarsal bursitis.

DISCUSSION

Morton's neuroma, also known as an interdigital neuroma, is a nonneoplastic perineural soft-tissue proliferation most commonly located at the level of the metatarsal heads, adjacent to the plantar digital nerves. The planter digital nerves are located in the distal intermetatarsal spaces and lie in close proximity to the intermetatarsal bursae and intermetatarsal ligaments. The neuroma is produced by a degenerative perineural fibrosing process occurring in and about the plantar digital nerve or nerves, probably resulting from repetitive microtrauma (1–3). It is thought that improperly fitted footwear, especially high-heeled shoes, results in increased stress on the soft tissue underlying the metatarsals, leading to the formation of an interdigital neuroma. The condition is much more common in women than in men, presumably as a result of their more restrictive foot wear. Morton's neuroma is most commonly located between the third and fourth intermetatarsals plantar to the metatarsal heads. They are also commonly found between the second and third intermetatarsals (4). Clinically, patients present with pain around the metatarsal heads that frequently radiates to the toes. The pain is exacerbated by walking and relieved by rest. Numbness of the forefoot may also be present (4,5).

Conventional radiographs and computed tomography are usually normal in patients with Morton's neuroma. On MR examination, Morton's neuroma can usually be visualized, particularly on contrast-enhanced images. However, very small neuromas may remain below the spatial resolving power of routine MR imaging. Morton's neuroma is best visualized on the coronal images of the forefoot as a small, oval, or rounded mass with somewhat ill-defined borders. The mass is located at the plantar aspect of the third or second intermetatarsal space, just plantar to the intermetatarsal ligament. The mass can extend dorsally into the intermetatarsal tissue and reach the dorsal aspect of the digit, forming a dumbbell-shaped appearance.

The typical Morton's neuroma is low to intermediate signal intensity on the T1-weighted sequence. On T2-weighted images, most interdigital neuromas demonstrate intermediate or very slightly increased signal intensity, owing to their densely packed fibrous tissue (2,4,5). The mass can be quite difficult to visualize on T2-weighted images because its signal intensity is similar to that of the adjacent soft tissues. On STIR sequences, the neuroma can show higher signal intensity than on the T2-weighted sequence. These signal characteristics help differentiate Morton's neuroma from a true neuroma, which almost always exhibits very high signal intensity on T2-weighted sequences. After the intravenous administration of gadolinium, Morton's neuroma enhances and can be better visualized than on nonenhanced sequences.

Morton's neuroma should be differentiated from fluid within the intermetatarsal bursa. The intermetatarsal bursae are located between the heads of the metatarsals and are most prominent at the second and third intermetatarsal spaces. The intermetatarsal bursa is located dorsal to the intermetatarsal ligament and proximal to the plantar digital nerves (2,3). Small amounts of fluid within the bursae are commonly found on MR imaging of the forefoot and are normal. Bursitis in this region produces a fluid collection that is located dorsal to the expected position of a neuroma. With isolated bursitis, contrast enhancement is not a prominent feature. One should be aware that Morton's neuroma can be associated with irritation and distention of the intermetatarsal bursa, so these two disorders may coexist. Distention of these bursae may be partly responsible for the pain that accompanies Morton's neuroma.

REFERENCES

1. Shankman S, Cisa J, Present D. Tumors of the ankle and foot. *Magn Reson Imaging Clin N Am* 1994;2:139–153.
2. Erickson SJ, Canale PB, Carrera GF, et al. Interdigital (Morton) neuroma: high-resolution MR imaging with a solenoid coil. *Radiology* 1991;181:833–836.
3. Steinbach LS. Painful syndromes around the ankle and foot: magnetic resonance imaging evaluation. *Top Magn Reson Imaging* 1998;9:311–326.
4. Zanetti M, Ledermann T, Zollinger H, et al. Efficacy of MR imaging in patients suspected of having Morton's neuroma. *AJR* 1997;168:529–532.
5. Terk MR, Kwong PK, Suthar M, et al. Morton neuroma: evaluation with MR imaging performed with contrast enhancement and fat suppression. *Radiology* 1993;189:239–241.

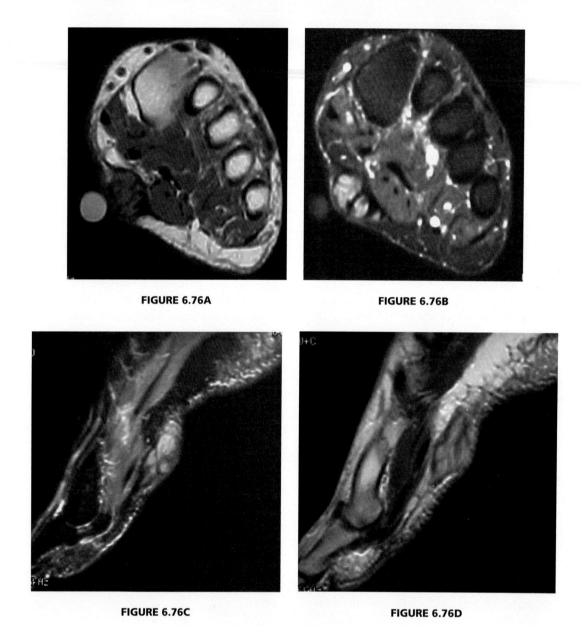

FIGURE 6.76A

FIGURE 6.76B

FIGURE 6.76C

FIGURE 6.76D

CLINICAL HISTORY

A young man felt a painless mass in the sole of his foot.

FINDINGS

The coronal T1-weighted image demonstrates a lobulated mass (Fig. 6.76A) in the subcutaneous fat, plantar to the base of the first metatarsal. The mass is low signal and mildly heterogeneous, with well-defined inferior and inferoposterior margins. Superiorly, the mass is intimately associated with the plantar fascia, which is displaced dorsally by the lesion. The corresponding fat-suppressed proton-density image (Fig. 6.76B) shows heterogeneous increased signal intensity within the lesion, with focal portions remaining low in signal. On the sagittal STIR image (Fig. 6.76C), the lesion is elongated with only moderately high signal intensity. The mass irregularly enhances on the sagittal fat-suppressed T1-weighted image obtained following intravenous contrast enhancement (Fig. 6.76D).

DIAGNOSIS

Plantar fibromatosis.

DISCUSSION

Plantar fibromatosis is a nonneoplastic but locally aggressive nodular overgrowth of fibrous tissue. Pathologically, the condition is characterized by the proliferation of fibroblasts in the subcutaneous tissue that replace portions of the plantar aponeurosis. The lesion is usually unencapsulated but well circumscribed. Growth is generally slow with local adherence to overlying skin and plantar fascia. Although the lesion is benign, it is frequently locally invasive, leading to high rates of incomplete resection (1–3). Since the lesions are unencapsulated, they can spread diffusely, resulting in recurrence rates as high as 75% after resection of the nodule (4).

The exact etiology of plantar fibromatosis is unknown. Traumatic, inflammatory, neurologic, degenerative, and familial causes have been suggested. An association of plantar fibromatosis with other sites of proliferation of fibrous tissue such as Duputytren's contractures of the hand, Peyronie's disease of the penis, and keloids is well documented (1,5,6). Plantar fibromatosis can be seen in all ages, though it is most common in middle-aged and elderly males. Patients are often asymptomatic. Mild pain and discomfort may be present after walking or prolonged standing. The most common complaint is the presence of a palpable mass or masses in the plantar soft tissues of the foot. The lesion can present as a solitary mass, as multiple nodules, or with bilateral lesions. The nodule most commonly arises near the anterior third and medial half of the plantar fascia. Rarely, the lesion extends dorsally into the plantar musculature.

Plantar fibromatosis is well shown on MR imaging. The mass or masses are located in the subcutaneous tissues of the foot, in association with the superficial surface of the medial portion of the plantar fascia. The inferior margins of the lesions are usually well circumscribed. The superior margins appear infiltrative and occasionally grow through the plantar fascia into the plantar muscles. On T1- and T2-weighted images, most lesions are heterogeneous but predominantly isointense or slightly brighter than muscle (1,5). The appearance on T2-weighted and STIR images is much more variable. The masses can remain dark or demonstrate areas of high signal intensity. Invasive lesions that remain low signal on the T2-weighted sequences can be difficult to distinguish from the musculature of the foot. After intravenous gadolinium injection, the masses show variable enhancement patterns. The majority of the lesions show marked enhancement, which helps to delineate the edges of the lesion from the adjacent soft tissues.

Submitted by Gerald Scidmore, Hoag Memorial Hospital, Newport Beach, CA.

REFERENCES

1. Resnick D, Kang HS. The ankle. In: Resnick D, Kang HS, eds. *Internal derangements of joints.* Philadelphia: WB Saunders, 1997:894–897.
2. Steinbach LS. Painful syndromes around the ankle and foot: magnetic resonance imaging evaluation. *Top Magn Reson Imaging* 1998;9:311–326.
3. Wu KK. Plantar fibromatosis of the foot. *J Foot Ankle Surg* 1994;33:98–101.
4. Pasternack WA, Davison GA. Plantar fibromatosis: staging by magnetic resonance imaging. *J Foot Ankle Surg* 1993;32:390–396.
5. Morrison WB, Schweitzer ME, Wapner KL, et al. Plantar fibromatosis: a benign aggressive neoplasm with a characteristic appearance on MR images. *Radiology* 1994;193:841–845.
6. Bruns BR, Hunter J, Yngve DA. Plantar fibromatosis. *Orthopedics* 1986;9:755–756.

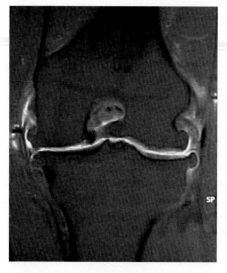

FIGURE 7.77A

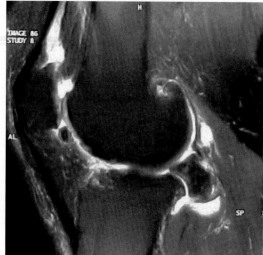

FIGURE 7.77C

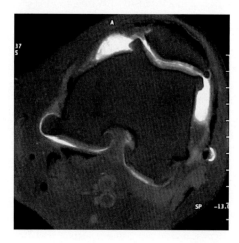

FIGURE 7.77B

CLINICAL HISTORY

This 50-year-old man with knee pain had a history of remote knee trauma.

FINDINGS

All the images are from fat-suppressed T1-weighted sequences obtained after intraarticular injection of gadolinium. The coronal (Fig. 7.77A) and axial (Fig. 7.77B) images show large marginal osteophytes on the femoral condyles, tibial plateaus, and patella. The subchondral bone is mildly irregular, as is the articular cartilage. Portions of the cartilage are completely denuded. The menisci are severely truncated. In addition, a large ossific density is present in the posterior joint (Fig. 7.77C), consistent with intraarticular body.

DIAGNOSIS

Advanced osteoarthritis of the knee.

DISCUSSION

Osteoarthritis, a degenerative disease of the joints, is the most common form of arthropathy. It results in degeneration and destruction of the articular cartilage and subchondral bone. Many factors predispose patients to degenerative joint disease. Aging is an important factor, owing to a diminished capacity of aging cartilage to resist mechanical stress. Under the age of 45, men tend to be affected more often than women. However, after the age of 45, women have a higher incidence of osteoarthritis than men. Obesity and nutritional and metabolic disorders are other factors associated with degenerative joint disease (1). Local trauma can also lead to degenerative joint disease.

Osteoarthritis is often divided into primary and secondary forms. The primary form affects all the weight-bearing joints, as well as the interphalangeal joints of the hands and feet. The exact cause of primary osteoarthritis is unknown. The secondary form is the result of a prior insult to the joints from trauma or other joint disease, such as infection, rheumatoid arthritis, or dysplasia. Other causes of secondary joint disease include crystal deposition, articular hemorrhage, acromegaly, and a host of other disorders.

Osteoarthritis is the most common type of arthropathy involving the knee and is commonly seen in patients with a history of prior injury, particularly following tears of the menisci or cruciate ligaments. The earliest sign is narrowing of the medial tibiofemoral compartment of the joint due to thinning and erosion of the cartilage. Subchondral sclerosis and osteophytosis of the medial tibiofemoral compartment subsequently develop. As the disease progresses, the tibia subluxes laterally and assumes a varus alignment relative to the femur. Subchondral sclerosis and cysts develop in the underlying bone as the cartilage is progressively damaged. Small fragments of cartilage or bone can become detached and form intraarticular bodies. The patellofemoral joint is affected to various degrees and has an appearance that is similar to that of the medial tibiofemoral joint. The lateral tibiofemoral joint remains normal until later in the disease process.

The diagnosis of osteoarthritis of the knee is usually on the basis of clinical examination, in conjunction with conventional radiographs. MR imaging can be helpful for further assessment of the joint, particularly the soft-tissue structures within and around the joints. Early cartilaginous changes, which cannot be identified on conventional radiographs, can be visualized with MR imaging. Gradient-echo sequences, conventional spin-echo, and fast spin-echo sequences have all been employed for the assessment of cartilage. We employ fat-suppressed proton-density fat spin sequences for routine assessment of cartilage, reserving the more time-consuming volumetric gradient-echo sequence for more specific cartilage assessment. On MR imaging, the normal hyaline cartilage has a trilaminar appearance, with low signal intensity within the most superficial layer, high signal intensity within the intermediate layer, and heterogeneous signal intensity within the innermost layer (2). The cause of this trilaminar appearance is a combination of the structure of cartilage and truncation artifacts from adjacent tissue interfaces (3). Loss of the trilaminar appearance of the cartilage can be seen in patients with early cartilage degeneration. Thinning and focal defects in the cartilage can also be seen with MR imaging. The use of intraarticular or intravenous gadolinium increases the sensitivity of MR for cartilage changes.

Focal subchondral bone marrow edema is often present in patients with advanced osteoarthritis. These areas show heterogeneously low signal on T1-weighted sequences and patchy areas of high signal on T2- or STIR-weighted sequences. The cause of the bone marrow edema underlying areas of cartilage damage is not well understood. Bone bruises due to microfractures from repetitive mechanical trauma, imbibition of joint fluid, and hyperemia from venous congestion have all been suggested (3). Subchondral sclerosis is not well shown on the MR images; however, osteophytes can be readily identified along the margin of the femoral condyle, tibial plateau, tibial spine, and patella. Subchondral cysts and geodes appear as well-defined, small, fluid-filled lesions in the subchondral bones.

REFERENCES

1. Brower AC. Osteoarthritis. In: Brower AC, eds. *Arthritis in black and white.* Philadelphia: WB Saunders, 1988:213–230.
2. Waldschmidt JG, Braunstein EM, Buckwalter KA. Magnetic resonance imaging of osteoarthritis. *Rheum Dis Clin North Am* 1999;25:451–465.
3. Resnick D. Degenerative diseases. In: Resnick D, eds. *Bone and joint imaging.* Philadelphia: WB Saunders, 1996:321–350.

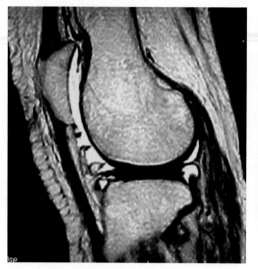

FIGURE 7.78A-1

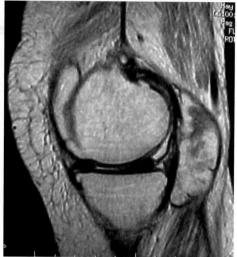

FIGURE 7.78B

CLINICAL HISTORY

An 81-year-old male had a swollen knee and patellar pain.

FINDINGS

A sagittal T2-weighted image demonstrates severe erosion of the patellar cartilage and remodeling of the subchondral bone of the patella (Fig. 7.78A-1). There is erosion of the distal femur (Fig. 7.78A-2, *arrow*) due to mechanical pressure from the patella. There are regions of low signal intensity in the synovial lining (Fig. 7.78A-2, *arrowhead*). On the sagittal proton-density-weighted image (Fig. 7.78B), there is thinning of the cartilage. Posterior to the medial femoral condyle is a large Baker's cyst containing heterogeneous signal.

DIAGNOSIS

Calcium pyrophosphate dihydrate crystal deposition disease.

DISCUSSION

Calcium pyrophosphate dihydrate (CPPD) crystal deposition disease is a common disorder that affects middle-aged and elderly individuals. It is the most common crystal-induced arthropathy (1,2). Patients with CPPD crystal deposition disease can be asymptomatic, have chronic progressive arthritis, or present with acute pseudogout. The disease can be hereditary, idiopathic, or associated with disorders such as hyperparathyroidism and hemochromatosis. It is characterized by the deposition of CPPD crystals in hyaline cartilage and fibrocartilage producing chondrocalcinosis. The CPPD crystals can also deposit in the synovium, capsule, tendons, and ligaments in and around the joints (1,3,4). Eight percent of patients with CPPD crystal deposition disease show chondrocalcinosis in the knee, and up to 75% show changes of pyrophosphate arthropathy (1).

CPPD arthropathy is a characteristic arthritis produced by the deposition of calcium pyrophosphate crystals. The vast majority of patients with pyrophosphate arthritis have radiographically evident chondrocalcinosis. The most commonly involved joints are the knee, pubic symphysis, and wrist (1,2). The involved joint space is narrowed, with subchondral sclerosis, osteophyte formation, and prominent subchondral cysts. In the knee, there is disproportionate involvement of the patellofemoral joint. A scalloped defect can be seen on the anterior femur due to abutment by the patella when the knee is extended. The relative lack of involvement of the femorotibial compartments helps differentiate CPPD arthropathy from conventional osteoarthritis.

Chondrocalcinosis can easily be overlooked on MR imaging. The small calcifications are often low signal and particularly difficult to recognize within the low-signal fibrocartilage of the menisci. Occasionally, intrameniscal high signal intensity may be present on T2-weighted spin-echo sequences, simulating the appearance of a meniscal tear. Although it is difficult to identify intrameniscal calcification, it has been reported that MR imaging is more sensitive than conventional radiographs for detecting hyaline cartilage calcification (5). In the hyaline cartilage, linear or punctuate areas of low signal may be noted, particularly on T2* gradient-echo sequences. These low-signal regions are thought to be due to calcific depositions within the cartilage. Pyrophosphate arthropathy can also be recognized by noting the disproportionate disease at the patellofemoral articulation.

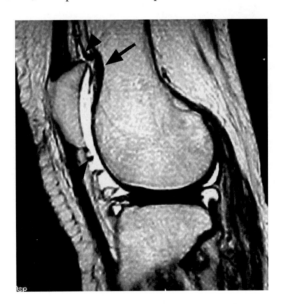

FIGURE 7.78A-2

REFERENCES

1. Resnick D. Calcium pyrophosphate dihydrate (CPPD) crystal deposition disease. In: Resnick D, ed. *Bone and joint imaging.* Philadelphia: WB Saunders, 1996:409–423.
2. Brower AC. Calcium pyrophosphate dihydrate (CPPD) crystal deposition disease. In: Brower AC, ed. *Arthritis in black and white.* Philadelphia: WB Saunders, 1988:271–280.
3. Ince A, Sundaram M. Calcium pyrophosphate dihydrate crystal deposition disease. *Orthopedics* 1996;19:80–81.
4. Yang BY, Sartoris DJ, Resnick D, et al. Calcium pyrophosphate dihydrate crystal deposition disease: frequency of tendon calcification about the knee. *J Rheumatol* 1996;23:883–888.
5. Beltran J, Marty-Delfaut E, Bencardino J, et al. Chondrocalcinosis of the hyaline cartilage of the knee: MRI manifestations. *Skeletal Radiol* 1998;27:369–374.

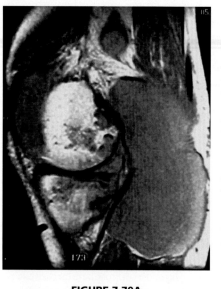

FIGURE 7.79A

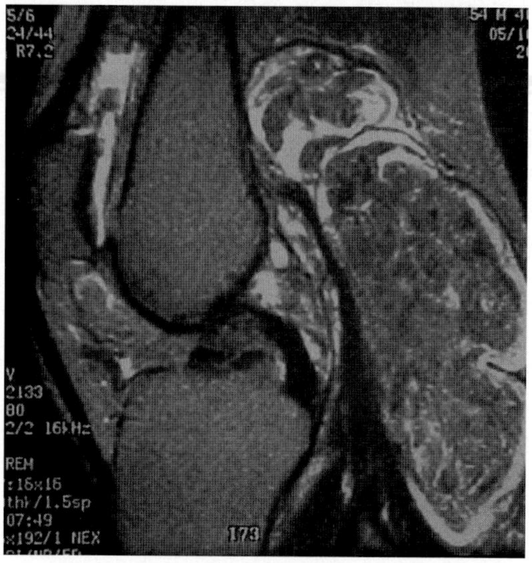

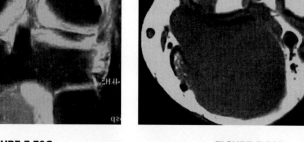

FIGURE 7.79B

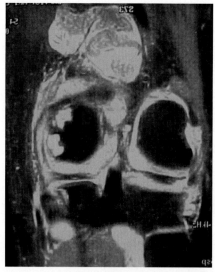

FIGURE 7.79C

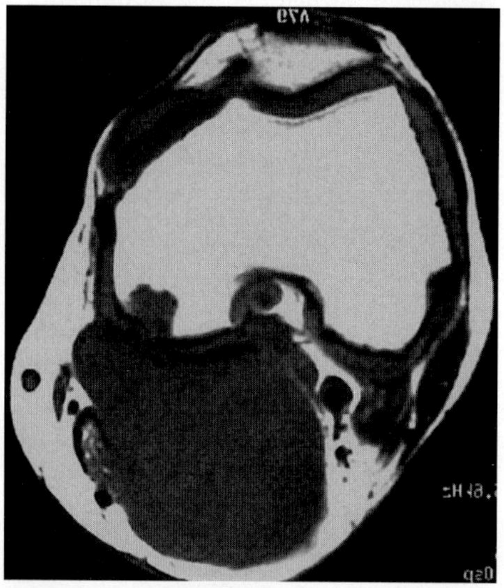

FIGURE 7.79D

CLINICAL HISTORY

A 54-year-old man with a known arthropathy complained of knee pain and swelling.

FINDINGS

On the sagittal proton-density-weighted image (Fig. 7.79A), the knee joint is distended with intermediate-signal-intensity material. Multiple areas of irregular bone erosion are present in both the femur and the tibia. A massive Baker's cyst is present. On the sagittal T2-weighted image (Fig. 7.79B), the joint distention is again seen. The material within the joint is heterogeneous, with multiple regions of low signal lining the joint and within the distended articu-

lation. The fat-suppressed coronal proton-density image (Fig. 7.79C) shows multiple erosions in the marginal regions of the joint. The multiple osseous erosions are associated with overlying defects in the cortical bone (Fig. 7.79A, 7.79C–D). The cartilage is thinned and eroded. The menisci are thinned and irregular, with a tear in the medial meniscus (Fig. 7.79A).

DIAGNOSIS

Rheumatoid arthritis of the knee joint with pannus and erosions.

DISCUSSION

Rheumatoid arthritis is a common polyarthritis with symmetric involvement of the synovial joints of the appendicular skeleton (1,2). Characteristic sites of involvement include the hands, feet, knees, hips, cervical spines, shoulders, and elbows. The disease is characterized by severe morning stiffness, swelling around the joints, painful articulations, and in some patients, subcutaneous nodules and systemic manifestations. Laboratory findings include a positive rheumatoid factor on serology and an elevated erythrocyte sedimentation rate.

Pathologically, typical rheumatoid lesions of the synovium and the soft tissue can be identified. Inflammatory changes occur in the synovium, which becomes edematous and hypertrophied with villous transformation. As the disease progress, there is invasion of the joint by the inflamed synovial pannus, a proliferative granulation tissue (3). Destruction of cartilage and bones is evident. Radiographically, typical findings include periarticular soft-tissue swelling and osteopenia, joint space narrowing, marginal bony erosions, effusion and synovial cyst formation, and joint malalignment.

Knee involvement is seen in 80% of patients with rheumatoid arthritis. Articular involvement is typically bilateral and symmetrical. Unlike osteoarthritis, the joint is uniformly narrowed due to diffuse cartilage loss in patients with rheumatoid arthritis. There is no noticeable reparative process, and therefore there is no evidence of osteophyte formation or subchondral sclerosis. Bony erosion may be present but is not as prominent as it is in the hands. Increased synovial fluid leads to distension of the joint by effusion. Large synovial cysts are often present, particularly in the form of a large Baker's cyst, which represents distention of the gastrocnemius-semimembranosus bursa. These large cysts frequently dissect down into the calf and are prone to rupture. Intraosseous synovial cysts and intraarticular rheumatoid nodules may be present (1,2).

MR imaging has been shown to be sensitive for diagnosis and evaluation of rheumatoid arthritis. MR imaging can detect pannus and bone erosion with greater sensitivity than conventional radiography. On T1-weighted images, collections of low signal intensity are seen within a distended joint. Some of this low-signal-intensity material represents pannus, and some is produced by articular effusion. On T1-weighted images, it is difficult to distinguish these two substances. On T2-weighted images, both pannus and fluid can show high signal intensity. Usually, pannus can be distinguished from fluid due to its more inhomogeneous appearance and the relatively lower signal of pannus caused by associated hemorrhage and fibrosis. Occasionally, it can be difficult to distinguish fluid from the pannus or synovial hypertrophy based solely on the T1- and T2-weighted images. Administration of intravenous gadolinium affords easy differentiation of pannus from effusion (3–5). The inflamed synovium and pannus demonstrate marked enhancement, whereas effusion remains low signal. The inflamed pannus has a characteristic lobulated frondlike appearance and is located at the periphery of the joint. MR is more sensitive for detection of small marginal erosions and subchondral cysts than the conventional radiographs (6). In one study, conventional radiographs detected only 12% of marginal erosions and 19% of subchondral cysts seen on MR images of the rheumatoid knee (6). Marginal erosions appear as areas of low signal intensity on T1-weighted images and as regions of heterogeneous high signal intensity on T2-weighted images. They tend to occur more frequently on the tibia than on the femur. The erosions are located in the marginal regions of the joint at the edges of the hyaline cartilage where the bone is exposed to the invading pannus.

Submitted by Dexter Witte, MidSouth Imaging and Therapeutics, Memphis, TN.

REFERENCES

1. Resnick D. Rheumatoid arthritis. In: Resnick D, ed. *Bone and joint imaging*. Philadelphia: WB Saunders, 1996:210–222.
2. Brower AC. Rheumatoid arthritis. In: Brower AC, ed. *Arthritis in black and white*. Philadelphia: WB Saunders, 1988:137–153.
3. Kursunoglu-Brahme S, Riccio T, Weisman MH, et al. Rheumatoid knee: role of gadopentetate-enhanced MR imaging. *Radiology* 1990;176:831–835.
4. Adam G, Dammer M, Bohndorf K, et al. Rheumatoid arthritis of the knee: value of gadopentetate dimeglumine-enhanced MR imaging. *AJR* 1991;156:125–129.
5. Konig H, Sieper J, Wolf K. Rheumatoid arthritis: evaluation of hypervascular and fibrous pannus with dynamic MR imaging enhanced with Gd-DTPA. *Radiology* 1990;176:473–477.
6. Poleksic L, Zdravkovic D, Jablanovic D, et al. Magnetic resonance imaging of bone destruction in rheumatoid arthritis: comparison with radiography. *Skeletal Radiol* 1993;22:577–580.

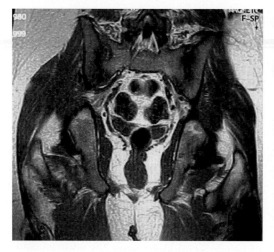

FIGURE 7.80A

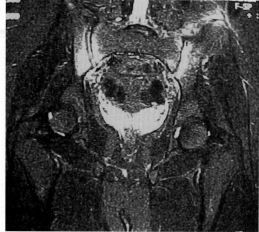

FIGURE 7.80B

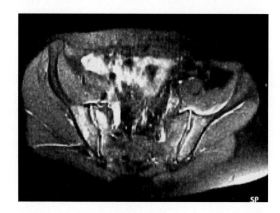

FIGURE 7.80C

CLINICAL HISTORY

An 18-year-old man had persistent lower back pain and heel pain.

FINDINGS

A coronal T1-weighted image of the pelvis shows ill-defined low signal intensity in the marrow adjacent to both sacroiliac joints (Fig. 7.80A). The articular surfaces are irregular and eroded. On the coronal STIR image (Fig. 7.80B) and the axial fat-suppressed proton-density-weighted image (Fig. 7.80C), high signal is present around both sacroiliac joints. The high signal extends into the adjacent iliacus muscle. Fluid is also present in the sacroiliac joints, which are irregular and appear widened.

DIAGNOSIS

Bilateral sacroiliitis due to ankylosing spondylitis.

DISCUSSION

The sacroiliac joint is composed of two portions. The posterior and superior portion of the joint is fibrous and is connected by intraosseous ligaments. The anterior and inferior one-half to two-thirds of the joint is a true synovial joint. The iliac articulating surface is covered by hyaline cartilage about 1 mm thick, whereas the sacral side is covered by fibrous cartilage, which is slightly thicker than the hyaline cartilage. Inflammatory sacroiliitis typically commences in the synovial portion of the joint and progresses to involve the entire joint. The synovial portion of the sacroiliac joint is the target site of a variety of inflammatory arthropathies (1). Sacroiliitis can be due to infection, ankylosing spondylitis, psoriatic arthritis, Reiter's syndrome, inflammatory bowel disease, and to a lesser extent, gout or rheumatoid arthritis.

Ankylosing spondylitis is a chronic autoimmune arthritis associated with the HLA-B27 antigen. The onset of the disease is typically in adolescents and there is a marked male predilection. The earliest sign of the disease is bilateral sacroiliitis, which is classically bilateral and symmetric (2). The absence of sacroiliitis essentially excludes the diagnosis of ankylosing spondylitis. The inflammatory process primarily involves the axial skeleton and then progresses to involve the large appendicular joints, particularly the hip and shoulder. Eventually ankylosis of the involved joints develops.

The initial symptoms of sacroiliitis are nonspecific, consisting of stiffness and the insidious onset of lower back pain. It is often difficult to distinguish inflammatory sacroiliitis from other causes of lower back pain based solely on history and physical examination (3,4). Diagnostic imaging plays an important role in the early diagnosis of ankylosing spondylitis. Conventional radiographs show osteopenia, joint space narrowing, and erosions. Sclerosis of the bone and ankylosis of the sacroiliac joint develop as the disease progresses (5).

Early diagnosis of sacroiliitis on conventional radiographs can be difficult due to the complex anatomy of the sacroiliac joints. Computed tomography, scintigraphy, and MR imaging have all been employed for assessment of the sacroiliac region. MR imaging has been shown to be highly sensitive for detecting sacroiliitis (3,4,6,7). Both coronal and axial images show the sacroiliac joints well, and the multiplanar capability of MR is very helpful for evaluating the complex curving articulation. The earliest finding of ankylosing spondylitis is loss of the normal thin band of intermediate-signal-intensity cartilage. Unfortunately, the cartilage in this area is difficult to visualize without high-resolution imaging. Erosions are found early in the course of the disease, particularly on the iliac side of the joint, where the cartilage is thinner and the bone is less protected. These erosions are surrounded by bone marrow edema, which can be very extensive and extend into the adjacent soft tissues. The edema is best seen with STIR or fat-suppressed T2-weighted images as regions of increased signal intensity in the sacral and iliac subchondral bone marrow. Both joint spaces widening and narrowing can be seen in patients with ankylosing spondylitis. With progressive disease, the joint narrows and ultimately fuses. Ankylosis is best appreciated on the T1-weighted MR images as a continuous band of marrow spanning the articulation. In the chronic phase of the disease, subchondral bone marrow edema resolves and is replaced by fibrosis of the marrow. The paraarticular marrow appears low signal intensity on both T1- and T2-weighted sequences due to fibrous tissue proliferation and remodeling of the damaged bone.

REFERENCES

1. Brower AC. Osteoarthritis. In: Brower AC, ed. *Arthritis in black and white.* Philadelphia: WB Saunders, 1988:103–104.
2. Brower AC. Osteoarthritis. In: Brower AC, ed. *Arthritis in black and white.* Philadelphia: WB Saunders, 1988:197–199.
3. Blum U, Buitrago-Tellez C, Mundinger A, et al. Magnetic resonance imaging (MRI) for detection of active sacroiliitis—a prospective study comparing conventional radiography, scintigraphy, and contrast enhanced MRI. *J Rheumatol* 1996;23:2107–2115.
4. Murphey MD, Wetzel LH, Bramble JM, et al. Sacroiliitis: MR imaging findings. *Radiology* 1991;180:239–244.
5. Resnick D. Ankylosing spondylitis. In: Resnick D, ed. *Bone and joint imaging.* Philadelphia: WB Saunders, 1996:246–249.
6. Hanly JG, Mitchell MJ, Barnes DC, et al. Early recognition of sacroiliitis by magnetic resonance imaging and single photon emission computed tomography [published erratum appears in *J Rheumatol* 1997;24:411–412. *J Rheumatol* 1994;21:2088–2095.
7. Docherty P, Mitchell MJ, MacMillan L, et al. Magnetic resonance imaging in the detection of sacroiliitis. *J Rheumatol* 1992;19:393–401.

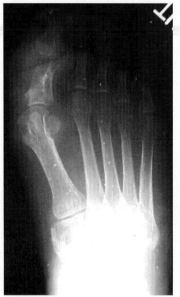

FIGURE 7.81A

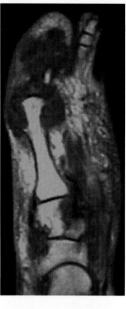

FIGURE 7.81B

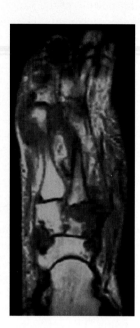

FIGURE 7.81C

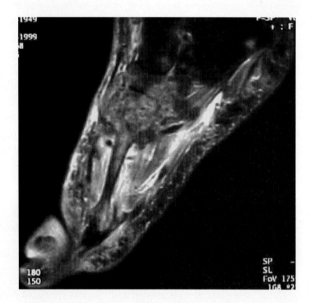

FIGURE 7.81D

CLINICAL HISTORY

An elderly man developed severe pain of the great toe.

FINDINGS

The frontal radiograph of the foot (Fig. 7.81A) shows large, well-defined periarticular erosions at the first metatarsophalangeal joint and first interphalangeal joint. Smaller erosions are present at the third and fifth metatarsal heads. Overhanging edges of proliferative bone are seen at the first metatarsophalangeal joint. There is soft-tissue swelling and increased soft-tissue density around the first metatarsophalangeal and interphalangeal articulations. On the axial T1-weighted images of the foot (Fig. 7.81B–C), there is a large amount of low- to intermediate-signal soft-tissue proliferation around the involved joints. Similar soft-tissue proliferation is present at the naviculocuneiform joint, as well as at the second and third tarsometatarsal joints. There are well-defined cortical erosions and extension of the soft-tissue material into the bone at these sites. On the sagittal STIR image (Fig. 7.81D), the soft-tissue masses show slightly increased signal intensity, with interspersed regions of low signal. Marrow edema is present adjacent to the osseous erosions. Extensive edema is seen in the dorsal and plantar soft tissue.

DIAGNOSIS

Tophaceous gout.

DISCUSSION

Gout is a crystal deposition disease producing an asymmetric polyarthritis. The disorder is the result of excessive production or decreased excretion of uric acid. Excess monosodium urate crystal deposits within the joints and in the soft tissue around the joints. The deposition of the urate crystal in the soft tissue results in tophus formation.

Gout has been classified into idiopathic gout and secondary gout caused by various disorders leading to hyperuricemia (1). Idiopathic gout is the most common form, affecting predominantly elderly men and less commonly, postmenopausal women. Gout has a predilection for lower-extremity involvement. The most common sites of gouty arthritis are the first metatarsophalangeal, intertarsal, tarsometatarsal, ankle, and knee articulations. The urate crystals incite an intense inflammatory reaction in the synovium. During acute gouty arthritis, patients experience the acute onset of severe pain, tenderness, and swelling of the affected joint. The attack can last for days to weeks. During an acute attack, large amounts of urate crystals can be aspirated from the joint. Patients then become asymptomatic until the next attack. During the chronic phase of gout, tophi deposit in the articular cartilage, subchondral bone, synovial membrane, joint capsule, tendons, ligaments, and bursae. These tophaceous deposits result in bone erosion and paraarticular osseous destruction (1,2).

Initial radiographs of patients with clinical symptoms of gout are usually unremarkable. Soft-tissue swelling may be seen during the acute attack, but erosions do not develop until the disease has been present for several years. In later stages of gout, after years of intermittent episodic arthritis, chronic tophaceous gout develops, producing well-defined erosions of the intraarticular or periarticular bones. The erosions are typically surrounded by a well-defined sclerotic margin and incite bone proliferation at their margin, resulting in an "overhanging edge" (1,2). When urate crystals deposit within the bone, intraosseous lytic lesions may be seen. Large tophi appear as dense soft-tissue masses adjacent to the joints. Uncommonly, calcifications may be seen in these tophaceous deposits.

MR imaging is not necessary for establishing the diagnosis of gout, which is usually established by aspiration of the joint. However, MR imaging is often obtained in patients with gout if the disorder is clinically unsuspected. The appearance of gout involving the foot has been well characterized on MR imaging. On MR, active gout shows soft-tissue edema around the affected joint. Fifty percent of patients have a prominent joint effusion. Bony erosions are also evident on the MR examinations. Bone marrow edema can be seen in most cases adjacent to the areas of osseous destruction. The most characteristic finding of gout is the identification of tophi. Tophi are isointense with muscle on T1-weighted images. On T2-weighted sequences, tophi exhibit variable signal intensity. The variation in T2 signal characteristics is thought to be due to differences in the calcium concentration within the tophaceous material. Tophi can show high signal intensity on T2-weighted images, but a low to intermediate heterogeneous pattern is much more common (3). After administration of intravenous gadolinium agent, tophi demonstrate near homogeneous enhancement. The adjacent synovium, tendon sheaths, ligaments, muscles, and bone marrow also enhance, because of the inflammatory response produced by the crystal deposition.

REFERENCES

1. Resnick D. Gouty arthritis. In: Resnick D, ed. *Bone and joint imaging*. Philadelphia: WB Saunders, 1996:396–405.
2. Surprenant MS, Levy AI, Hanft JR. Intraosseous gout of the foot: an unusual case report. *J Foot Ankle Surg* 1996;35:237–243.
3. Yu JS, Chung C, Recht M, et al. MR imaging of tophaceous gout. *AJR* 1997;168:523–527.

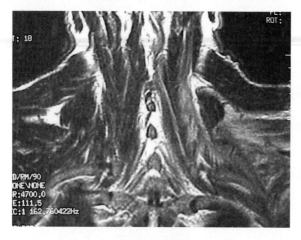

FIGURE 8.82A

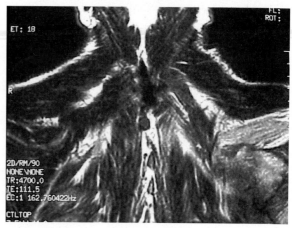

FIGURE 8.82B

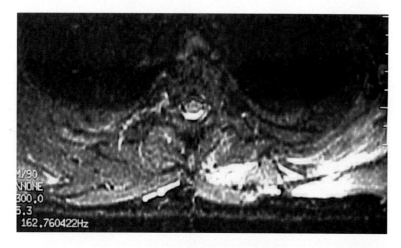

FIGURE 8.82C

CLINICAL HISTORY

A 62-year-old man complained of severe weakness in his left arm following a motor vehicle accident 4 weeks previously, at which time he sustained a brachial plexus injury.

FINDINGS

Coronal proton-density and T2-weighted images of the posterior paraspinal region (Fig. 8.82A–B) show muscle asymmetry, with diminution in size of the paraspinal musculature on the left side in the cervicothoracic region. There is also abnormal increased signal within the left paraspinal muscles, particularly within the supraspinatus muscles (Fig. 8.82B). The muscle asymmetry and abnormal signal are even more apparent on the axial short tau inversion recovery (STIR) image (Fig. 8.82C).

DIAGNOSIS

Denervation of muscle with muscle edema related to recent brachial plexus injury.

DISCUSSION

On MR imaging, normal skeletal muscle has a longitudinal striated appearance, with interlaced linear regions of fat within and between the major muscle bundles. Normal muscle is low signal on all sequences, is symmetric in size, and has a feathery appearance due to its interspersed fat.

Acutely denervated muscle shows a paucity of findings on MR imaging. MR signal alterations are usually seen several weeks following the loss of neural innervation (1,2). In subacute denervation, the MR examination shows high signal on T2-weighted and inversion recovery sequences within the denervated muscles. These signal changes are thought to be due to an increased amount of extracellular water in the damaged muscle (2). Typically, the size of the muscle remains normal or is slightly diminished. Uncommonly, denervated muscle in the lower extremity can undergo hypertrophy and appear as a mass lesion (3). The MR appearance of muscle edema within a muscle of normal size is nonspecific and is similar to the changes associated with muscle injury, inflammatory myositis, muscle infarction, pyomyositis, and peritumoral edema. Clinical history and the distribution of the muscle abnormalities, which correspond to a specific nerve distribution, allow accurate diagnosis of muscle denervation (1). With brachial plexus injury, signal changes within the cervical and upper thoracic paraspinal musculature, as well as in the involved arm muscles, are most prominent (4,5). Traction injuries of the brachial plexus produce most pronounced alterations in the posterior paraspinal musculature and proximal shoulder girdle muscles (5).

In chronic denervation, the changes of muscle edema resolve, and the involved muscles undergo significant volume loss and fatty atrophy. At this stage of denervation, increased intramuscular fat is the most prominent finding on MR imaging. The presence of fatty change in chronically denervated muscle suggests an irreversible lesion (2).

REFERENCES

1. Uetani M, Hayashi K, Matsunaga N, et al. Denervated skeletal muscle: MR imaging. *Radiology* 1993;189:511–515.
2. Fleckenstein JL, Watumull D, Conner KE, et al. Denervated human skeletal muscle: MR imaging evaluation. *Radiology* 1993;187:213–218.
3. Petersilge CA, Pathria MN, Gentili A, et al. Denervation hypertrophy of muscle: MR features. *JCAT* 1995;19:596–600.
4. Sallomi D, Janzen DL, Munk PL, et al. Muscle denervation patterns in upper limb nerve injuries: MR imaging findings and anatomic basis. *AJR* 1998;171:779–784.
5. Uetani M, Hayashi K, Hashmi R, et al. Traction injuries of the brachial plexus: signal intensity changes of the posterior cervical paraspinal muscles on MRI. *JCAT* 1997;21:790–795.

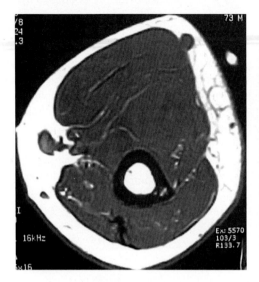

FIGURE 8.83A

FIGURE 8.83B

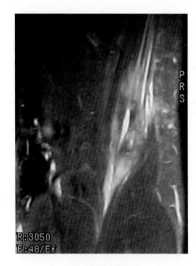

FIGURE 8.83C

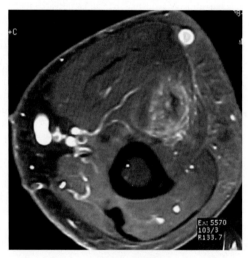

FIGURE 8.83D

CLINICAL HISTORY

A 73-year-old man injured his arm during a vigorous game of golf 3 weeks prior to this MR examination. Physical examination revealed weakness on active elbow flexion.

FINDINGS

The axial T1-weighted image (Fig. 8.83A) of the upper arm has isointense signal within the brachialis muscle. On the T2-weighted image, the same region has abnormal increased signal on both the axial (Fig. 8.83B) and the coronal (Fig. 8.83C) images. Despite the abnormal signal alter-

ations, the muscle morphology appears relatively preserved and there is no mass effect on the adjacent vessels and subcutaneous tissues. The coronal image shows longitudinally oriented streaks of increased signal intensity within the brachialis muscle. Maximal signal abnormality is located at the level of the myotendinous junction of the brachialis. There is intratendinous edema and thickening of the fibers of the brachialis tendon at the myotendinous junction. An axial fat-suppressed T1-weighted image (Fig. 8.83D) obtained following intravenous contrast enhancement shows strandy peripheral enhancement in the area of muscle abnormality.

DIAGNOSIS

Grade 2 strain of the brachialis muscle.

DISCUSSION

Muscle injuries related to a single episode of severe trauma are subdivided into muscle strain and muscle contusion, depending on the mechanism of injury. The term *strain* is applied to muscle trauma, whereas the term *sprain* is reserved for injury to the ligaments. A muscle strain is caused by an indirect injury, whereas a muscle contusion is due to direct nonpenetrating concussive trauma to the muscle (1). The MR appearance of a strain is similar to that of a contusion, but the clinical history and the location of the typical muscle strain differ from that of muscle contusion. Contusions often produce more extensive muscle injury than the typical sprain and are more likely to be associated with extensive hemorrhage within the muscle. Without adequate clinical history, it can be difficult to distinguish these two forms of muscle trauma.

Muscle strains typically involve the myotendinous junction of the muscle, where the muscle fibers interdigitate directly to the fibers of the tendon (1). The myotendinous junction is particularly vulnerable to injury because it is the structurally weakest region in the myotendinous unit due to its limited capacity for energy absorption (2). Muscle strain is most commonly seen involving the long fusiform muscles of the lower extremity, particularly those muscles that cross two articulations. Muscles that contain a high proportion of type 2 fibers and perform predominantly eccentric contraction are at particularly high risk for exertional injury (1,2). The most common sites of muscle strain are the biceps brachii, rectus femoris, semimembranosus, and medial gastrocnemius (2).

The severity of muscle strain depends on the duration of stress loading as well as the rate and magnitude of stress applied to this region (2). Strains are subdivided into three grades by orthopedic surgeons. A grade 1 strain is the mildest form of muscle injury. Patients with a grade 1 strain have mild edema and hemorrhage within the muscle but suffer no weakness or loss of function. A grade 2 strain is a moderately severe injury associated with weakness of the injured muscle, but muscle function is still maintained. The most severe form of muscle strain, the grade 3 injury, produces weakness and loss of function of the injured muscle. Loss of function can be permanent following a severe muscle injury.

On MR imaging, a grade 1 strain demonstrates normal muscle morphology and only mild abnormalities of muscle signal, particularly in the region of the myotendinous junction. Typically, the T1-weighted images remain entirely normal and signal alterations are only evident on the T2 or STIR images (3). The areas of high signal extend from the myotendinous junction into the adjacent muscle fibers, tracking along the fascicles in a feathery pattern (2). In grade 2 strains, there are signal changes and mild alterations in the muscle morphology. The T2-weighted images show irregularity, thinning, and mild waviness of the tendon fibers. Muscle edema and hemorrhage are more prominent, often collecting in the subfascial regions around the injured muscle (3). More significant morphologic alterations are present in the grade 3 strain, which represents a complete rupture of the myotendinous junction. Large amounts of hemorrhage may be present, obscuring the anatomy and making it difficult to distinguish a complete myotendinous disruption from a high-grade partial tear (2). The diagnosis is obvious if the tendon ends are retracted, producing a gap in the soft tissues at the expected position of the myotendinous junction and allowing the muscle to bunch up away from the region (2).

REFERENCES

1. Steinbach LS, Fleckenstein JL, Mink JH. Magnetic resonance imaging of muscle injuries. *Orthopedics* 1994;17:991–999.
2. Palmer WE, Kuong SJ, Elmadbouh HM. MR imaging of myotendinous strain. *AJR* 1999;173:703–709.
3. Fleckenstein JL, Weatherall PT, Parkey RW, et al. Sports related muscle injuries: evaluation with MR imaging. *Radiology* 1989;172:793–798.

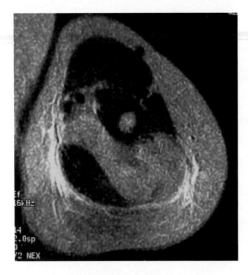 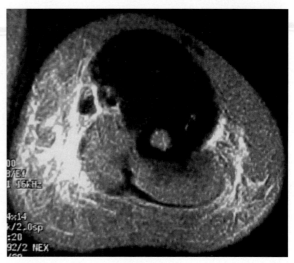

FIGURE 8.84A　　　　　　　　　　**FIGURE 8.84B**

CLINICAL HISTORY

A 48-year-old woman complained of 2 days of severe arm pain. She had been lifting weights in the gym 4 days prior to this MR examination.

FINDINGS

A heavily T2-weighted axial image (Fig. 8.84A) of the upper arm shows abnormal signal within the triceps muscle. The muscle does not appear enlarged. A more caudal image (Fig. 8.84B) from the same series again shows the abnormal signal within the triceps muscle. There is increased signal within the subcutaneous tissues, and small collections of subfascial fluid are present adjacent to the abnormal muscle. The muscle appeared normal on the T1-weighted images (not shown).

DIAGNOSIS

Delayed-onset muscle soreness.

DISCUSSION

Exercise can be followed by pain, muscle soreness, and muscle swelling, particularly in the deconditioned individual (1,2). Muscle pain developing in healthy individuals hours or days following exercise has been termed *delayed-onset muscle soreness* (DOMS) (1). Unlike the acute onset of symptoms during exercise associated with a muscle strain, the symptoms of DOMS develop gradually 1 to 2 days following exercise, progressively increase to peak 2 to 3 days following the activity, and then spontaneously resolve after approximately 1 week (1).

During exercise, muscle can perform eccentric (muscle-lengthening) or concentric (muscle-shortening) contractions. DOMS is most likely to occur following exercise associated with eccentric muscle contractions (3). Eccentric actions involve forced active muscle lengthening or stretching and are the primary cause of both acute and chronic exertional muscle injury (3). Eccentric contractions have lower oxygen requirements, less lactate production, and fewer activated motor units than concentric contractions of the muscle (4). However, eccentric contractions result in more force developing within the muscle than with comparable concentric exercise, leading to overuse injury of the muscle (3).

DOMS is linked to ultrastructural muscle damage and increased plasma levels of muscle enzymes such as creatine kinase (2). The microscopic muscle damage associated with DOMS results in increased muscle edema and increased interstitial fluid that produce signal abnormalities on MR imaging (5). The appearance of DOMS is similar to the muscle abnormalities seen in patients with a mild muscle strain, so a patient's history is required to make an accurate diagnosis of DOMS. On T1-weighted images, mild enlargement of the muscle may be present. The presence and degree of muscle enlargement correlate with elevations of serum creatine kinase (2). Despite a quantitative increase in the T1 relaxation time of the muscle in DOMS, T1-weighted images typically show minimal signal alteration within the damaged muscle. Increased signal is seen within the injured muscle on the T2-weighted and STIR images (3,5). The muscle architecture remains preserved and the edema parallels the orientation of the muscle fascicles. Signal changes and clinical symptoms are maximal in the region of the myotendinous junction of the muscle. Subcutaneous edema and small perifascial fluid collections can be seen in the early phase of the injury (5). Although the clinical symptoms typically resolve quickly, the MR signal changes of DOMS have been reported to persist for up to 80 days following exercise (3).

REFERENCES

1. Steinbach LS, Fleckenstein JL, Mink JH. Magnetic resonance imaging of muscle injuries. *Orthopedics* 1994;17:991–999.
2. Evans GF, Haller RG, Wyrick PS, et al. Submaximal delayed-onset muscle soreness: correlations between MR imaging findings and clinical measures. *Radiology* 1998;208:815–820.
3. Shellock FG, Fukunaga T, Mink JH, et al. Exertional muscle injury: evaluation of concentric versus eccentric actions with serial MR imaging. *Radiology* 1991;179:659–664.
4. Shellock FG, Fukunaga T, Mink JH, et al. Acute effects of exercise on MR imaging of skeletal muscle: concentric vs eccentric actions. *AJR* 1991;156:765–768.
5. Fleckenstein JL, Weatherall PT, Parkey RW, et al. Sports related muscle injuries: evaluation with MR imaging. *Radiology* 1989;172:793–798.

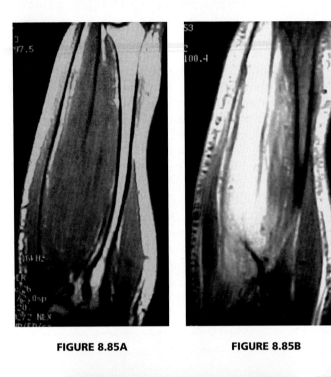

FIGURE 8.85A

FIGURE 8.85B

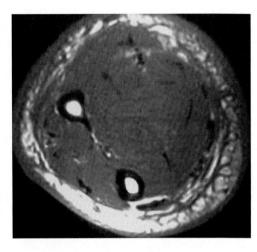

FIGURE 8.85C

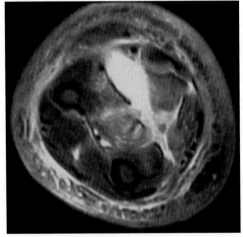

FIGURE 8.85D

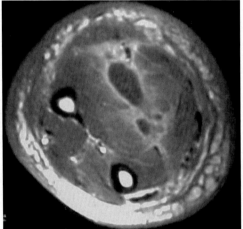

FIGURE 8.85E

CLINICAL HISTORY

A 32-year-old male with AIDS developed a mild fever and complained of severe pain and swelling of his forearm.

FINDINGS

Sagittal T1-weighted (Fig. 8.85A) and STIR (Fig. 8.85B) images of the forearm show thickening of the volar forearm muscles and increased signal extending through-out the forearm musculature on the STIR image. The axial T1-weighted image (Fig. 8.85C) shows enlargement of the volar muscles, loss of the intramuscular fat planes, and subcutaneous stranding. On the axial T2-weighted image (Fig. 8.85D), extensive signal abnormality is present within the muscle, and there is edema in the subcutaneous tissues. The fat-suppressed T1-weighted axial image obtained after contrast enhancement (Fig. 8.85E) shows an irregular area of fluid that does not enhance, surrounded by a high-signal-intensity enhancing rim. The underlying bone is normal.

DIAGNOSIS

Pyomyositis and soft-tissue abscess.

DISCUSSION

Pyomyositis is a primary bacterial infection that develops within skeletal muscle (1). Pyomyositis is also termed *tropical pyomyositis* because it has traditionally been a disease encountered in patients living in hot and humid climates. Historically, pyomyositis has been rare in the United States. Recently, there has been a significant increase in the incidence of this condition, largely because of the increased incidence of this serious infection among patients with AIDS (1). Although advanced AIDS represents the most significant risk factor for pyomyositis in this country, other disorders associated with primary muscle infection include diabetes mellitus, corticosteroid use, underlying malignancy, connective-tissue disease, and varied hematologic diseases (1). The most common causative organism is *Staphylococcus aureus,* which accounts for 90% of cases of pyomyositis.

Pyomyositis is typically limited to one extremity, though multiple muscles may be involved within that extremity. Multiple sites of muscle involvement are present in almost half of patients (2). Unlike autoimmune polymyositis, which is also seen with increased frequency in patients with AIDS, the muscle involvement in pyomyositis is asymmetric and not associated with weakness of the involved musculature (2). The large muscles of the lower extremity, particularly the muscles of the buttock and thigh, are most frequently involved. Adjacent soft-tissue inflammation may be present, but subcutaneous inflammatory changes are minimal compared with those seen in patients with cellulitis or fasciitis and are disproportionately less prominent than the muscular abnormalities (2). The underlying bony cortex and bone marrow are typically not involved (3).

MR imaging is the modality of choice for diagnosis and assessment of deep soft-tissue infection. In the early stages of pyomyositis, the infected muscle is enlarged and shows changes of muscle edema and inflammation on MR imaging. As the infection progresses, muscle necrosis is common, leading to the development of fluid collections related to myonecrosis and abscess formation in the soft tissue (1). On T1-weighted MR, findings are minimal except for subcutaneous edema and mild enlargement of the affected muscles due to increased volume of interstitial fluid and fluid collections. High signal is seen within the muscle on MR on T2-weighted images. Pyomyositis is commonly associated with intramuscular abscess formation (1–3). The signal characteristics of soft-tissue abscesses are highly variable on MR. The typical abscess is a round or oval mass that is low signal on T1-weighted images and high signal on T2-weighted images. The highly proteinaceous material within a chronic abscess can appear high or intermediate in signal intensity on T1-weighted images. High-signal material is seen most commonly at the periphery of an abscess, forming a prominent high signal rim at the margin of the abscess (2). The exact etiology of the high-signal rim remains uncertain; some investigators speculate that it may be related to paramagnetic material at the edge of the abscess (1). On T1-weighted images obtained following contrast enhancement, the thick, irregular wall of the abscess enhances avidly, whereas the central region of the abscess remains low in signal.

REFERENCES

1. Gordon BA, Martinez S, Collins AJ. Pyomyositis: characteristics at CT and MR imaging. *Radiology* 1995;197:279–286.
2. Fleckenstein JL, Burns DK, Murphy FK, et al. Differential diagnosis of bacterial myositis in AIDS: evaluation with MR imaging. *Radiology* 1991;179:653–658.
3. Steinbach LS, Tehranzedah J, Fleckenstein JL, et al. Human immunodeficiency virus infection: musculoskeletal manifestations. *Radiology* 1993;186:833–838.

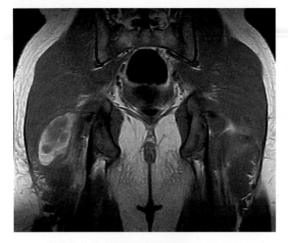

FIGURE 8.86A

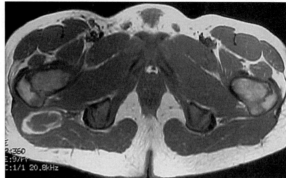

FIGURE 8.86B

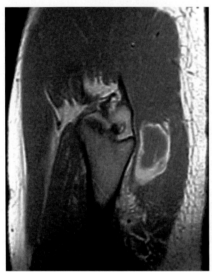

FIGURE 8.86C

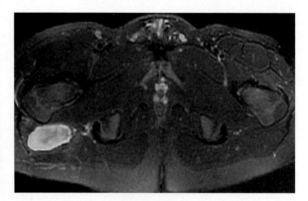

FIGURE 8.86D

CLINICAL HISTORY

A 13-year-old boy fell 1 week ago and complained of buttock tenderness and fullness.

FINDINGS

The T1-weighted coronal (Fig. 8.86A), axial (Fig. 8.86B), and sagittal (Fig. 8.86C) images of the pelvis show a 5-cm oval mass within the right gluteus maximus muscle. The mass is well defined, with a high-signal peripheral rim and low-signal material in its center. The underlying bone is normal. On the axial T2-weighted image (Fig. 8.86D), the entire mass appears high in signal, with slight internal inhomogeneity. There is no fluid-fluid level within the lesion. The adjacent soft tissues appear normal.

DIAGNOSIS

Buttock hematoma within the gluteus maximus muscle.

DISCUSSION

Soft-tissue hemorrhage can be due to penetrating trauma, muscle strain, blunt injury, coagulopathy, or underlying vascular malformation, or it can occur within a necrotic soft-tissue neoplasm (1). Trauma is the most common cause of soft-tissue hemorrhage, particularly in the young patient. Hemorrhage is most commonly due to indirect traumatic strain or direct contusion by blunt trauma. Soft-tissue hemorrhage can take one of two forms in the mesenchymal tissues. Parenchymal hemorrhage refers to blood that dissects through the stromal tissues in an ill-defined, feathery pattern. Alternatively, the bleeding can be more focal and confined, forming a discrete collection known as a hematoma (2). Unlike parenchymal hemorrhage, a hematoma has little or no interspersed stromal tissue. Hematomas are frequently surrounded by regions of parenchymal hemorrhage, and these two forms often coexist. It has been shown that the evolution of soft-tissue bleeding is different in these two forms of hemorrhage and that only the hematoma shows the distinctive MR signal characteristics of blood breakdown (2).

Hematomas can be seen within the muscle, in the intermuscular fat planes, or within the subcutaneous tissues. The diagnosis is usually obvious in posttraumatic cases because of the history of recent injury. Although the diagnosis is not difficult in these cases, other patients do not provide a history of an injury. In such patients, the MR findings are frequently diagnostic of a collection of blood due to the characteristic appearance of blood in some of its intermediate phases of breakdown. The MR appearance of a hematoma is highly variable, depending upon the stage of breakdown of the blood produced within the collection. In general, the MR appearance of soft-tissue hematoma follows the same evolution as that of hematoma in the brain, though the progression of blood breakdown in soft tissue is often slower and less predictable (2,3).

Blood passes through a number of stages as it evolves.

Hyperacute hematoma of the musculoskeletal tissues is rarely imaged with MR. When the hematoma first develops, it has a unique appearance because of the presence of intracellular deoxyhemoglobin, resulting in low signal on both T1- and T2-weighted images (4). Acute hematoma has a nonspecific appearance of low signal on T1-weighted and high signal on T2-weighted images. Fluid-fluid levels may be seen in large hematomas, indicating their liquid nature.

Subacute hematomas are collections of blood that are at least 3 to 4 days old (2,3). As the hematoma ages, ferrous iron containing hemoglobin is oxidized to methemoglobin, which contains ferric iron (3). *In vitro*, the maximal conversion to methemoglobin takes place at 80 to 90 hours (3). Methemoglobin has a distinctive appearance on MR because it produces T1 shortening, resulting in high signal within the hematoma on T1-weighted images. In general, this methemoglobin effect is most prominent at the periphery of the hematoma. (2) Hemorrhagic neoplasms typically show the most methemoglobin in the center of the lesion because bleeding takes place in areas of central necrosis. Over time, the entire hematoma can contain methemoglobin and appear uniformly high in signal.

Eventually, the methemoglobin within the hematoma is resorbed or degrades. Some of the iron in the methemoglobin is converted to hemosiderin and ferritin, which deposit in the hemorrhage and adjacent tissues (4). Hemosiderin and ferritin are closely related chemically and are characteristic of a chronic hematoma (4). These substances result in signal loss on both T1- and T2-weighted images, producing a low-signal halo around the hematoma. Gradient-echo sequences show the presence of hemosiderin and ferritin to best advantage due to the magnetic susceptibility artifact produced by these substances. Over time, as the methemoglobin degrades, the entire hematoma contracts and appears low signal.

REFERENCES

1. Steinbach LS, Fleckenstein JL, Mink JH. Magnetic resonance imaging of muscle injuries. *Orthopedics* 1994;17:991–999.
2. Swenson SJ, Keller PL, Berquist TH, et al. Magnetic resonance imaging of hemorrhage. *AJR* 1985;145:921–927.
3. Unger EC, Glazer HS, Lee JKT, et al. MRI of extracranial hematomas: preliminary observations. *AJR* 1986;146:403–407.
4. Gamori JM, Grossman RI. Mechanisms responsible for the MR appearance and evolution of intracranial hemorrhage. *Radiographics* 1988;8:427–440.

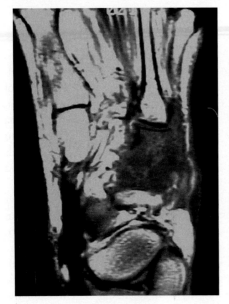

FIGURE 9.87A

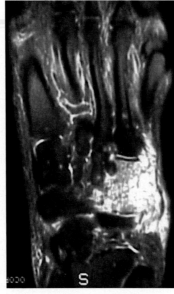

FIGURE 9.87B

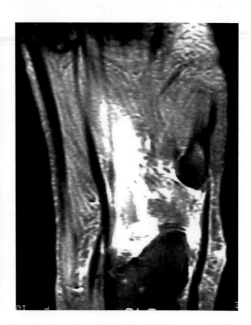

FIGURE 9.87C

CLINICAL HISTORY

A 34-year-old woman with a long-standing history of vasculitis and chronic skin infections developed severe pain in her foot.

FINDINGS

The axial T1-weighted image (Fig. 9.87A) of the foot shows loss of the normal high marrow signal within the cuboid. The corresponding fat-suppressed T2-weighted image (Fig. 9.87B) shows intense signal increase within the bone. The lateral cortical border of the cuboid is very irregular, with multiple areas of cortical destruction. Abnormal increased signal is also present in the adjacent soft tissues. Following intravenous gadolinium enhancement, a more plantar image (Fig. 9.87C) shows mild enhancement within the bone and intense enhancement in the soft tissues adjacent to the cuboid. Enhancement of soft tissue throughout the plantar region is also present.

DIAGNOSIS

Osteomyelitis of the cuboid.

DISCUSSION

The term *osteomyelitis* refers to infection of the bone marrow. The most common causative organism in all age groups is *Staphylococcus aureus*. In the infant, group D streptococcus and staphylococci are the major causative agents. The three major mechanisms responsible for infection of the bone marrow are hematogenous dissemination, direct spread from adjacent soft-tissue infection, and direct inoculation of the bone through a skin ulcer or penetrating wound. In children, osteomyelitis due to hematogenous spread is most common and typically affects the metaphyseal regions of the femur and tibia. The childhood metaphysis is involved due to the slow, looping blood supply adjacent to the physeal plate. Osteomyelitis in the adult is less common than that in the child. Adult osteomyelitis is more likely to be associated with soft-tissue abscesses and pathologic fractures than that in children. In adults, hematogenous osteomyelitis typically involves the axial skeleton, which still contains vascular active hematopoietic marrow. Osteomyelitis due to penetrating wounds is most common in the hands and feet due to their vulnerability to penetration and the superficial locations of the bones in these regions.

MR imaging plays an important role in detecting osteomyelitis, determining the extent of the infection, identifying associated soft-tissue abscess formation, planning surgical debridement, and monitoring antibiotic therapy (1). MR is as sensitive as scintigraphy for detection of acute osteomyelitis but has higher specificity and provides more anatomic information than the bone scan (2). Osteomyelitis produces marrow inhomogeneity with poorly defined regions of low signal marrow on T1-weighted sequences that show increases in signal intensity on T2-weighted or short tau inversion recovery (STIR) images and that typically enhance following intravenous administration of gadolinium (3,4). The cortical bone appears normal in the acute phases of osteomyelitis, though periostitis is often present very early in the course of the disease (5). As the infection becomes more established, areas of cortical destruction and reactive changes of cortical thickening and irregularity become apparent. Edema in the adjacent noninfected bone and the periosseous soft tissues is a prominent feature on MR imaging. MR can overestimate the extent of infection due to difficulty in distinguishing adjacent reactive edema from frank marrow infection.

REFERENCES

1. Gold Rh, Hawkins RA, Katz RD. Bacterial osteomyelitis: findings on plain radiography, CT, MR, and scintigraphy. *AJR* 1991;157:365–370.
2. Morrison WB, Schweitzer ME, Bock GW, et al. Diagnosis of osteomyelitis: utility of fat-suppressed contrast-enhanced MR imaging. *Radiology* 1993;189:251–257.
3. Quinn SF, Murray W, Clark RA, et al. MR imaging of chronic osteomyelitis. *J Comput Assist Tomogr* 1988;12:113–117.
4. Dangman BC, Hoffer FA, Rand FF, et al. Osteomyelitis in children: gadolinium-enhanced MR imaging. *Radiology* 1992;182:743–747.
5. Erdman WA, Ramburro F, Jayson HT, et al. Osteomyelitis: characteristics and pitfalls of diagnosis with MR imaging. *Radiology* 1991;180:533–539.

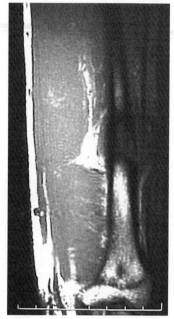

FIGURE 9.88A

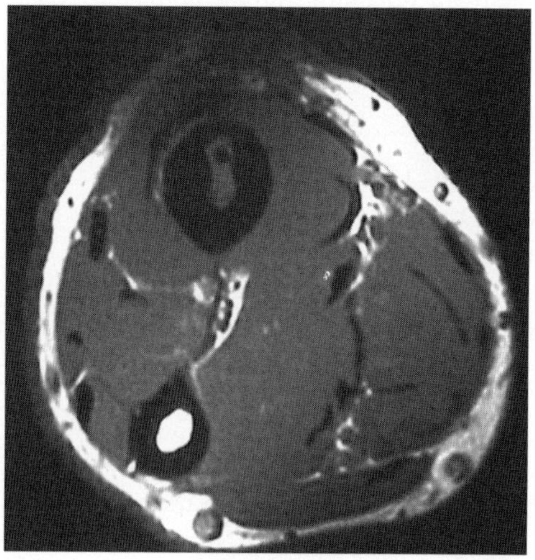

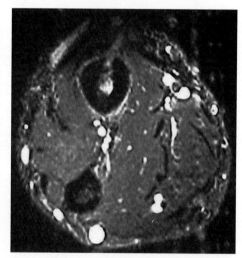

FIGURE 9.88B

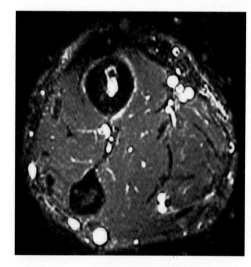

FIGURE 9.88C

FIGURE 9.88D

CLINICAL HISTORY

A male intravenous drug abuser complained of persistent skin drainage at the level of his mid-forearm.

FINDINGS

A coronal T1-weighted image of the forearm (Fig. 9.88A) shows a 3-cm area of marrow replacement in the midradius. The low-signal lesion has ill-defined margins, and there is cortical thickening overlying and adjacent to the area of marrow abnormality. A thin low-signal linear structure is present within the lateral portion of the lesion. Axial T1-weighted

(Fig. 9.88B) and fat-suppressed proton-density-weighted (Fig. 9.88C) images show the small, isolated, low-signal fragment of bone, completely isolated from the remainder of the bone by soft tissue. An adjacent fat-suppressed proton-den-sity-weighted axial image reveals a defect in the radial side of the cortex (Fig. 9.88D). Both of the axial images show a thin circumferential zone of high signal surrounding the bone produced by periosteal proliferation.

DIAGNOSIS

Chronic osteomyelitis of the radius with intraosseous sequestrum and cortical cloaca.

DISCUSSION

Osteomyelitis is traditionally classified into acute, sub-acute, and chronic stages. These stages are not clearly defined and typically overlap. Chronic active osteomyelitis can produce a variety of osseous and soft-tissue abnormalities. One of the most characteristic features of active chronic osteomyelitis is the formation of a sequestrum within the bone at the site of the infection. A sequestrum is a fragment of necrotic bone that is completely isolated from the normal living bone by a layer of purulent material, infected tissue, and granulation tissue (1). The typical sequestrum is a small, longitudinally oriented fragment arising from the original osseous cortex. The size of an intraosseous sequestrum is variable, though the area of necrotic bone is rarely more than a few centimeters in length, and most are considerably smaller. The sequestered bone is not attached to the viable bone and is devascularized, making it difficult to treat the infection with systemic antibiotics. The sequestrum therefore acts as a nidus of infection that is very difficult to sterilize without surgical removal. An area of chronic osteomyelitis may contain more than one such fragment.

Other bony lesions that are associated with chronic osteomyelitis include the involucrum and the cloaca (1). An involucrum represents a layer of living bone that surrounds the dead osseous fragment. A cloaca is an opening within an involucrum and is a site of drainage of pus and granulation tissue. The purulent material draining outside the bone via the cloaca often produces a small focal abscess on the surface of the bone. Sinus tracks can develop so that the purulent material draining from the bone via the cloaca can subsequently drain to the skin (2).

A sequestrum can be difficult to identify with conventional radiography, particularly if the fragment is small and there is extensive reactive sclerosis in the adjacent bone. The necrotic linear bone fragment is denser than the adjacent bone and surrounded by a thin zone of soft tissue that separates it from the rest of the bone. Computed tomography is extremely helpful for identifying these necrotic fragments. Sequestered bone can be identified on MR imaging, and this modality has the advantage of multiplanar imaging, which is very helpful for confirming that the bone fragment is truly isolated from the remaining bone (3). The necrotic sequestrum itself remains low signal on all MR imaging sequences. The surrounding infected soft tissue is dark on the T1-weighted images and increases in signal on the T2-weighted images. Occasionally, a zone of high signal is seen at the periphery of the chronic intraosseous infection, produced by highly vascularized granulation tissue containing thick-walled arterioles (4). Contrast between the sequestrum and adjacent soft tissues is poor on the T1-weighted images. The sequestered bone is best visualized on either proton-density or T2-weighted images through the site of infection. Cloaca within the cortex are a common accompaniment and are best seen on the T2-weighted images. Cortical thickening and periostitis are also features of chronic osteomyelitis (5). Periostitis surrounding an area of chronic osteomyelitis can be seen on the T2-weighted images, particularly those obtained in the axial plane. The periosteal proliferation produces a thin zone of high signal that circumferentially surrounds the bone cortex.

REFERENCES

1. Resnick D. Osteomyelitis, septic arthritis, and soft tissue infection: the mechanisms and situations. In: Resnick D, Niwayama G, eds. *Diagnosis of bone and joint disorders,* 2nd ed. Philadelphia: WB Saunders, 1988:2524–2618.
2. Mason MD, Zlatkin MB, Esterhai JL, et al. Chronic complicated osteomyelitis of the lower extremity: evaluation with MR imaging. *Radiology* 1989;173:355–359.
3. Quinn SF, Murray W, Clark RA, et al. MR imaging of chronic osteomyelitis. *J Comput Assist Tomogr* 1988;12:113–117.
4. Grey AC, Davies AM, Mangham DC, et al. The "penumbra sign" on T1-weighted MR imaging in subacute osteomyelitis: frequency, cause and significance. *Clin Radiol* 1998;53:587–592.
5. Cohen MD, Cory DA, Kleiman M, et al. Magnetic resonance differentiation of acute and chronic osteomyelitis in children. *Clin Radiol* 1990;41:53–56.

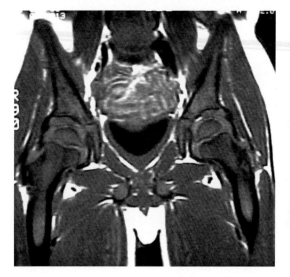 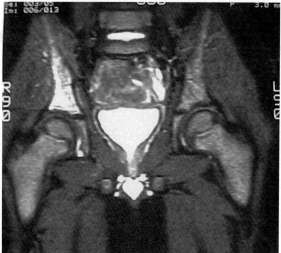

FIGURE 9.89A　　　　　　　　　　**FIGURE 9.89B**

CLINICAL HISTORY

A 3-year-old boy with a known bone marrow disorder developed an acutely painful left hip.

FINDINGS

A T1-weighted coronal image of the pelvis and proximal femora (Fig. 9.89A) shows very-low-signal marrow within the pelvic bones, as well as within the epiphyses of the proximal femora. The marrow appears isointense to the skeletal muscle. No expansion of the bone is present. The coronal STIR image (Fig. 9.89B) shows a large area of abnormal increased marrow signal in the right acetabulum. There is no effusion in the adjacent hip joint, and the periarticular soft tissues are normal. The remainder of the marrow remains low signal on this sequence.

DIAGNOSIS

Sickle cell disease with expanded hematopoietic marrow and acute infarction of the right acetabular marrow.

DISCUSSION

Sickle cell disease is an inherited defect in hemoglobin synthesis resulting in the formation of a low solubility beta-hemoglobin. The sickle cell gene is present in 8% of the black population, and 0.15% to 0.2% of blacks are homozygous for the gene defect, resulting in sickle cell disease (1). The marrow of patients with sickle cell disease appears abnormal on MR imaging for a variety of reasons. The abnormal hemoglobin undergoes "sickling" under conditions of low oxygen tension, resulting in vascular compromise and widespread microinfarction of the bone marrow. Chronic hemolysis of the abnormal red cell constituents results in a continuous demand for hematopoiesis, leading to hyperplasia of the red marrow. In addition, chronic hemolysis results in hemosiderin deposition within the bone marrow. Secondary hemosiderosis is a well-recognized complication of sickle cell disease and contributes to the diffuse loss of marrow signal, particularly on gradient-echo sequences.

Expansion of the hematopoietic marrow is a common feature of sickle cell disease (2). Hematopoietic expansion is a symmetric generalized process. The expanded red marrow decreases the overall signal of the marrow on both T1- and T2-weighted pulse sequences. The normal marrow should be higher signal than the muscle on T1-weighted sequences because of the admixture of fat with the normal marrow elements (3). In the patient with sickle cell disease, the proportion of marrow fat is diminished, resulting in low-signal marrow due to the preponderance of red marrow. The presence of abnormal marrow is easiest to appreciate in the normally fatty epiphyses and apophyses of the axial skeleton. In the normal child, low-signal marrow should never be present in the proximal femoral epiphyses past infancy (4).

Osteonecrosis of bone is a common complication due to the vascular compromise produced by the sickled cells. Infarcts are most common in the subchondral and metadiaphyseal regions of the long bones, though any bone in the skeleton can develop osteonecrosis in patients with sickle cell disease. Multiple infarcts of varying ages are commonly present. Acute infarcts appear as areas of marrow edema, showing low signal on T1-weighted images that increases in signal on T2 weighting (2). In patients with sickle cell disease, particularly young children with large amounts of hematopoietic marrow, osteonecrosis can be very difficult to recognize on T1-weighted images because of the lack of contrast between the low-signal infarcted marrow and the background low-signal hematopoietic marrow. In the young child with acute marrow infarction, T2-weighted or inversion recovery sequences show increased marrow signal and are more sensitive than the T1-weighted images.

Differentiation of sickle cell infarction from osteomyelitis is difficult during the acute phase, prior to the development of the characteristic low-signal bands and rings of established osteonecrosis. The patient with sickle cell disease has an increased risk for osteomyelitis, which is often caused by enteric organisms released into the bloodstream by microinfarctions of the bowel wall. Correlation with the clinical symptoms and physical examination, white cell count, response to hydration and oxygenation, and imaging features are essential. Radionuclide imaging can be very useful for distinguishing aspectic infarction from osteomyelitis of the bone. In some cases, needle aspiration is required to distinguish these two entities.

REFERENCES

1. Sebes JI. Diagnostic imaging of bone and joint abnormalities associated with sickle cell hemoglobinopathies. *AJR* 1989;152:1153–1159.
2. Rao VM, Fishman M, Mitchell DG, et al. Painful sickle cell crisis: bone marrow patterns observed with MR imaging. *Radiology* 1986;161:211–215.
3. Pathria MN, Isaacs P. Magnetic resonance imaging of bone marrow. *Curr Opin Radiol* 1992;4:21–31.
4. Jaramillo D, Laor T, Hoffer FA, et al. Epiphyseal marrow in infancy: MR imaging. *Radiology* 1991;180:809–812.

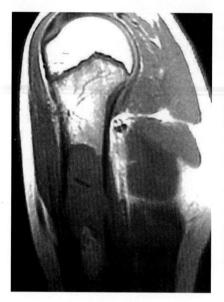 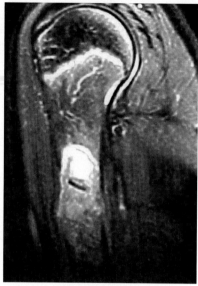 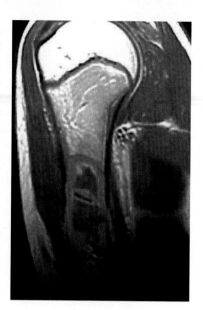

FIGURE 9.90A   **FIGURE 9.90B**   **FIGURE 9.90C**

CLINICAL HISTORY

A 14-year-old heard a snap and had severe upper arm pain after a minor fall.

FINDINGS

The oblique coronal T1-weighted (Fig. 9.90A) and T2-weighted (Fig. 9.90B) images of the right proximal humerus show a central metadiaphyseal lesion mildly expanding the bone. The lesion is low signal on the T1-weighted images and shows inhomogeneous increase in signal on T2 weighting. There is cortical disruption of both the medial and the lateral humeral cortex. Following intravenous contrast enhancement with gadolinium, the oblique coronal fat-suppressed T1-weighted image shows enhancement at the periphery of the lesion (Fig. 9.90C). Centrally, there is a thin linear fragment that remains low signal on all the imaging sequences, though there is enhancement surrounding the fragment on the contrast-enhanced image.

DIAGNOSIS

Fracture of unicameral bone cyst with central "fallen fragment sign."

DISCUSSION

The unicameral bone cyst (UBC), also known as a simple bone cyst, is a common benign lesion of the growing skeleton, representing up to 5% of primary bone lesions (1). The majority of lesions are found in children and adolescents; the majority of UBCs are located in either the proximal humerus or the proximal femur of children and adolescents (2). Clinically, these cystic lesions are typically asymptomatic unless complicated by pathologic fracture, which complicated the course of the lesions in approximately 65% of cases (1). Following such a fracture, the lesions often heal uneventfully. Treatment with intralesional corticosteroid injection has been employed for lesions that are symptomatic or that fail to involute spontaneously or following a fracture (3).

Radiographically, the typical appearance of a UBC is that of a mildly expansile, well-defined lytic lesion in the metadiaphyseal region of a long bone. When the cyst fractures, fragments of cortical bone that become displaced within the fluid-filled cavity of the lesion settle to the dependent portions of the cyst, giving rise to the appearance of the "fallen fragment sign" (1).

The appearance of a UBC on both computed tomography and MR imaging is that of a well-defined central zone of fluid signal surrounded by a thin zone of bone sclerosis (3,4). On MR imaging, the thin cellular lining of the cyst can be seen at the periphery of the lesion following enhancement with intravenous gadolinium. This enhancing lining often appears thicker and more prominent in lesions detected in adulthood (5). When the cyst has been complicated by a fracture, the internal characteristics become inhomogeneous because of admixture of fluid and blood. The central spicule of bone, produced by a cortical fragment displaced into the fluid center of the lesion, remains low signal on all sequences and is pathognomonic of a UBC complicated by fracture.

REFERENCES

1. Killeen KL. The fallen fragment sign. *Radiology* 1998;207:261–262.
2. Blumberg ML. CT of iliac unicameral bone cysts. *AJR* 1981;136:1231–1232.
3. Fernbach SK, Blumenthal DH, Poznanski AK, et al. Radiographic changes in unicameral bone cysts following direct injection of steroids: a report of 14 cases. *Radiology* 1981;140:689–695.
4. Abdelwahab IF, Hermann G, Lewis MM, et al. Case report 534: simple bone cyst of the acetabulum and ischium. *Skeletal Radiol* 1989;18:157–159.
5. Ehara S, Nishida J, Shiraishi H, et al. Eccentric simple bone cysts of the femoral neck in adults. *Clin Imaging* 1997;21:233–236.

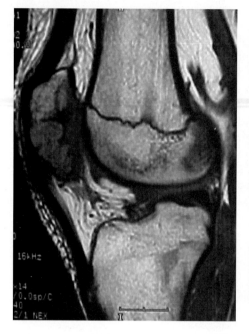

FIGURE 9.91A

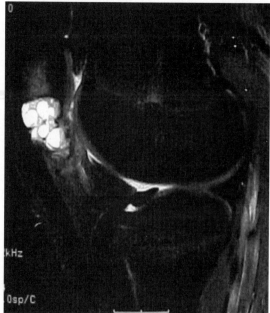

FIGURE 9.91B

CLINICAL HISTORY

A 15-year-old boy complained of 3 months of patellar discomfort.

FINDINGS

The T1-weighted sagittal image (Fig. 9.91A) shows an expansile low-signal, tumorlike lesion in the inferior pole of the patella. The lesion is well marginated and the overlying cortex is thinned but intact. The internal signal is inhomogeneous, with regions of intermediate signal intensity. On the sagittal fat-suppressed heavily T2-weighted image (Fig. 9.91B), the lesion increases in signal intensity. Multiple fluid-fluid levels are present within the region of abnormal marrow.

DIAGNOSIS

Aneurysmal bone cyst of the patella.

DISCUSSION

An aneurysmal bone cyst (ABC) is a benign but locally aggressive lytic lesion of bone of unknown etiology. ABCs are most commonly located eccentrically in the metaphyseal region of the long bones in children, teenagers, and young adults (1). The lesion, which has a tendency to be markedly expansile, consists of multiple blood-filled thin-walled cavities that lack a normal endothelial lining (2). ABC can develop as a primary bone lesion or it can develop secondarily adjacent to another bony disorder, particularly when that disorder results in alterations of local osseous hemodynamics. Secondary ABCs have been associated with underlying Paget's disease, giant cell tumor, fibrous dysplasia, fracture, and a host of other bone lesions (3).

Radiographs of ABC demonstrate marked osseous expansion and cortical thinning overlying the lesion. The thin shell of the remaining cortex may be difficult to identify on radiographs, though it can usually be seen with computed tomography (CT). CT can also show the presence of fluid-fluid levels within the lesion if the slices are obtained perpendicular to their orientation (4). The finding of fluid-fluid levels within an expansile lesion has been emphasized as a rather specific indicator of an ABC, particularly when septations within the lesion result in multiple levels. The MR findings of ABC are even more specific than CT due to the ability of MR to demonstrate the internal constituents of the lesion (5). The fluid-fluid levels in an ABC are produced by layering of serum and blood products, and therefore can show a wide spectrum of signal characteristics, depending on the stage of breakdown of the blood products (5). Fluid-fluid levels are not pathognomonic of an ABC, having also been described in osteomyelitis, telangiectatic osteosarcoma, giant cell tumor, and many other lesions of bone.

Submitted by Joel Rubenstein, Reno, NV.

REFERENCES

1. Cory DA, Fritsch SA, Cohen MD, et al. Aneurysmal bone cysts: imaging findings and embolotherapy. *AJR* 1989;153:369–373.
2. Munk PL, Helms CA, Holt RG, et al. MR imaging of aneurysmal bone cysts. *AJR* 1989;153:99–101.
3. Dagher AP, Magid D, Johnson CA, et al. Aneurysmal bone cyst developing after anterior cruciate ligament tear and repair. *AJR* 1992;158:1289–1291.
4. Hudson TM. Fluid levels in aneurysmal bone cysts: a CT feature. *AJR* 1984;141:1001–1004.
5. Beltran J, Simon DC, Levy M, et al. Aneurysmal bone cysts: MR imaging at 1.5 T. *Radiology* 1986;158:689–690.

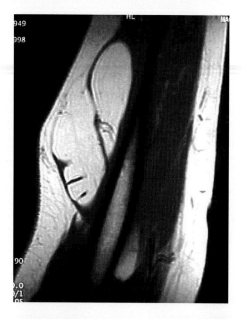

FIGURE 9.92A

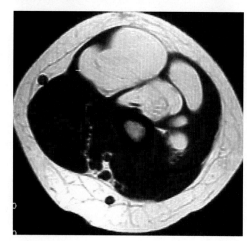

FIGURE 9.92B

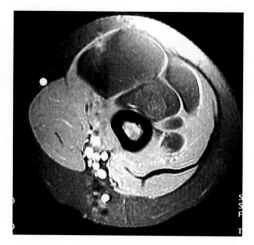

FIGURE 9.92C

CLINICAL HISTORY

A 50-year-old woman complained of pain and an enlarging mass in her upper arm.

FINDINGS

The sagittal T1-weighted image shows a large, well-defined, lobulated, intramuscular, soft-tissue mass anterolateral to the humeral shaft (Fig. 9.92A). A T1-weighted axial image obtained in the midportion of the lesion shows that although the mass is predominantly high signal, a few thin, low-signal septations are present within the lesion (Fig.

9.92B). The axial fat-suppressed T1-weighted image obtained following intravenous gadolinium enhancement (Fig. 9.92C) shows that the signal within the mass has decreased, similar to subcutaneous fat, and that there is no capsular or septal enhancement.

DIAGNOSIS

Soft-tissue lipoma.

DISCUSSION

Lipomas are the most common benign soft-tissue neoplasm. Patients with lipoma are typically middle-aged or elderly and present with a mass that is typically slow growing and relatively painless for its size (1). Although the classic lipoma is composed of mature adipose tissue, numerous histologic variants of this lesion have been described that contain vessels, fibrous tissue, neural elements, and other nonadipose tissues (1). Lipomas can also be characterized as either superficial or deep, with the superficial variant being more common (1).

The diagnosis of lipoma is easy to establish with CT and MR imaging when the lesion is composed largely of mature fat. Lipomas are well-defined, lobulated, homogeneous lesions that are best seen on the T1-weighted images, particularly if they are deep within the musculature. Subcutaneous lipomas can be difficult to differentiate from the normal high-signal subcutaneous fat. On MR imaging, the signal of fat varies according to the pulse sequence employed (2,3). On T1-weighted imaging, the lipoma shows high signal, paralleling the signal of subcutaneous fat. On T2-weighted images, the signal from fat decreases to intermediate. Fat-suppression and STIR sequences can be used to decrease the signal within the lesion and help confirm the presence of fatty tissue (3). The typical lipoma does not show any significant enhancement with gadolinium, though small amounts of enhancement within the thin capsule and septae within the lesion should be considered normal.

The most difficult lesion to differentiate from lipoma is well-differentiated liposarcoma. Although most liposarcomas are of the myxoid variety and therefore appear low signal on T1-weighted imaging, approximately 10% to 25% of malignant fatty lesions are the well-differentiated variant of liposarcomas and consist primarily of mature fat (4). Liposarcoma can usually be differentiated from lipoma by the presence of signal inhomogeneity, peripheral soft-tissue nodularity, thick septae, and intralesional necrosis. Other than lipoma and liposarcoma, soft-tissue lesions that can be bright on T1-weighted MR imaging include hemangioma, subacute hemorrhage within a tumor, subacute traumatic hematoma, and paramagnetic substances within the patient (1,2).

REFERENCES

1. Kransdorf MJ, Moser RP, Meis JM, et al. Fat-containing soft-tissue masses of the extremities. *Radiographics* 1991;11:81–106.
2. Dooms GC, Hricak H, Sollitto RA, et al. Lipomatous tumors and tumors with fatty component: MR imaging potential and comparison with MR and CT results. *Radiology* 1985;157:479–483.
3. Munk PL, Lee MJ, Janzen DL, et al. Lipoma and liposarcoma: evaluation using CT and MR imaging. *AJR* 1997;169:589–594.
4. Jelinek JS, Kransdorf MJ, Shmookler BM, et al. Liposarcoma of the extremities: MR and CT findings in the histological subtypes. *Radiology* 1993;186:455–459.

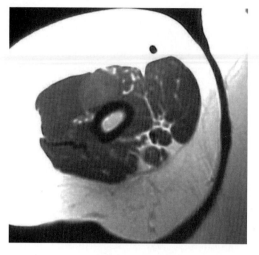

FIGURE 9.93A

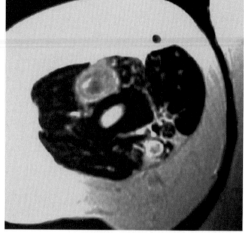

FIGURE 9.93B

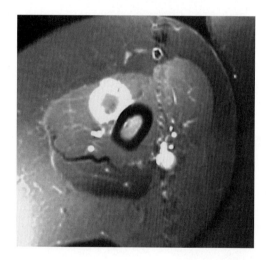

FIGURE 9.93C

CLINICAL HISTORY

A 37-year-old woman discovered a painless mass in her upper arm.

FINDINGS

The T1-weighted axial image (Fig. 9.93A) shows a subtle low-signal mass anterolateral to the humerus. The underlying bone appears normal. On the T2-weighted image (Fig. 9.93B), the mass appears well defined and demonstrates a "target" appearance, with a low-signal center and a high-signal perimeter. A fat-suppressed T1-weighted image obtained following intravenous gadolinium administrations (Fig. 9.93C) shows intense enhancement at the periphery of the lesion and persistence of a low-signal central region.

DIAGNOSIS

Peripheral localized neurofibroma.

DISCUSSION

Neurogenic neoplasms account for approximately 10% of all benign soft-tissue tumors. Benign neurogenic neoplasms of the soft tissues include neurofibroma, neurilemoma (schwannoma), nerve sheath ganglion, Morton's neuroma, and posttraumatic neuroma (1). Soft-tissue neurofibromas are the most common form of neural tumor found in the soft tissues. These benign tumors arise from peripheral nerve sheath and are most common in young adults. Unlike schwannomas, resection of a neurofibroma entails sacrificing the involved nerve as the latter is inseparable from the normal neural elements (2).

Neurofibromas are classified into three types: localized, diffuse, and plexiform. All three forms can be found in patients with neurofibromatosis, though only the plexiform form is consistently associated with that syndrome. The solitary localized form is most common, representing approximately 90% of all neurofibromas, and the vast majority of patients with a neurofibroma have no stigmata of generalized neurofibromatosis (1). Diffuse neurofibroma is less well defined and more infiltrative than the localized form, whereas the plexiform variant is typically much longer and larger, and has a more tortuous form, resembling a "bag of worms" (1).

Localized neurofibromas are slow-growing lesions and are therefore typically smaller than 5 cm in diameter at diagnosis. The lesions tend to be fusiform and have a "tail" at the site of the entering and exiting nerve. The diagnosis of neurofibroma can often be made when the soft-tissue mass is along the distribution of a peripheral nerve and appears to be connected to the nerve at its proximal and distal ends (2). On MR imaging, localized neurofibromas are well-defined, homogeneous lesions that appear low signal on T1-weighted sequences. A majority of neurofibromas demonstrate a central region of diminished signal on T2-weighted images, surrounded by a peripheral zone of high signal (2,3). This "target" appearance has been emphasized as a reliable feature of a benign neurofibroma on MR imaging. The low-signal central region is produced by T2 shortening caused by the dense collagen and fibrous tissue present in the central regions of a neurofibroma (2). The target sign may be absent when there is cystic degeneration, hemorrhage, or necrosis within the center of a benign neurofibroma (3). Neurofibrosarcoma also lacks the characteristic target sign of a benign localized neurofibroma (4). Malignant degeneration to neurofibrosarcoma is an uncommon complication of neurofibroma that is strongly suggestive of underlying neurofibromatosis (4).

REFERENCES

1. Murphey MD, Smith WS, Smith SE, et al. Imaging of musculoskeletal neurogenic tumors: radiologic-pathologic correlation. *Radiographics* 1999;19:1253–1280.
2. Suh J, Abenoza P, Galloway HR, et al. Peripheral (extracranial) nerve tumors: correlation of MR imaging and histologic findings. *Radiology* 1992;183:341–346.
3. Varma DGK, Moulopoulos A, Sara AS, et al. MR imaging of extracranial nerve sheath tumors. *J Comput Assist Tomogr* 1992;16:448–453.
4. Bhargava R, Parham DM, Lasater OE, et al. MR imaging differentiation of benign and malignant peripheral nerve sheath tumors: use of the target sign. *Pediatr Radiol* 1997;27:124–129.

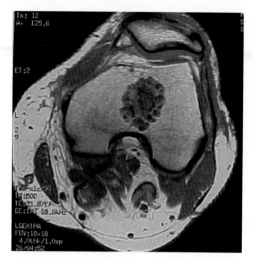

FIGURE 9.94A

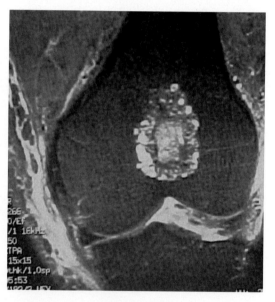

FIGURE 9.94B

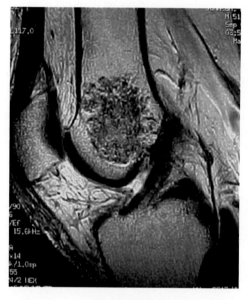

FIGURE 9.94C

FIGURE 9.94D

CLINICAL HISTORY

A 51-year-old male had knee radiographs following an injury. MR was requested to evaluate a tumor of the distal femur incidentally noted on the radiographs.

FINDINGS

An axial T1-weighted image of the distal femur shows a multilobulated mass located centrally in the medullary cavity (Fig. 9.94A). Following gadolinium enhancement, the fat-suppressed T1-weighted image (Fig. 9.94B) shows enhancement of the peripheral portions of the lobules in a "rings and arcs" pattern. The sagittal T2-weighted image

(Fig. 9.94C) shows persistent low signal within the lesion. The coronal fat-suppressed proton-density-weighted image (Fig. 9.94D) again shows the inhomogeneous signal within the tumor, with multiple rounded lobular densities forming the periphery of the mass. There is also soft-tissue edema and an effusion related to the recent injury to the knee.

DIAGNOSIS

Enchondroma of the distal femur.

DISCUSSION

Enchondroma is a benign intramedullary neoplasm made up of mature cartilage. It is one of the most common neoplasms of the adult skeleton, accounting for up to 17% of all benign skeletal tumors (1). The most common location of enchondroma is within the small bones of the hand, particularly the diaphyseal and metadiaphyseal regions of the metacarpals and phalanges. When enchondroma is identified within the bones of the hands, the lesion is easily recognized and additional imaging is rarely indicated (2). In the remainder of the skeleton, the appendicular bones are much more frequent sites of enchondroma than the axial skeletal structures (1). The imaging features of enchondroma in the long or flat bones of the skeleton are less definitive, and additional imaging is often required to establish a specific diagnosis.

Enchondroma is often detected as an incidental finding on radiographic imaging obtained for some other reason (2). Large lesions can produce enough local pressure within the bone to become painful. Pathologic fracture through an enchondroma is another common mode of presentation, particularly with lesions in the small bones of the hand (3). The most serious complication related to enchondroma is transformation to malignant chondrosarcoma. Patients with this dreaded complication develop increased pain, enlargement of the enchondroma, resorption of mineralization within the lesion and adjacent bone lysis, as well as soft-tissue extension of the lesion (1).

Enchondroma is typically a monostotic lesion. Multiple enchondromatosis (Ollier disease) and the association of multiple enchondromata with soft-tissue hemangiomas (Maffucci syndrome) are uncommon but well-recognized syndromes that present at a younger age and have a much higher risk for complications related to the cartilage lesions.

Malignant transformation of enchondroma into chondrosarcoma has been reported to occur in up to 1% of patients with monostotic enchondroma and up to 10% to 15% of patients with Ollier disease or Maffucci syndrome (4).

The growth pattern of the low-grade intramedullary cartilaginous lesions is classically lobulated (3). Enchondromas show peripheral lobulation, as well as multiple small round and oval intralesional lobules uniformly distributed throughout the lesion. These lobules vary from 3 to 15 mm in diameter, reflecting the typical growth pattern of cartilage. Calcification at the margins of the lobules produces the classic "rings and arcs" of mineralization seen on radiographs and CT (3). On MR imaging, the lobular growth pattern of cartilage is also readily apparent. Multiple rounded areas of cartilage are present within the lesion, and the margin of the enchondroma is very well defined. The signal within the lesion parallels that of hyaline cartilage, with low signal intensity on T1-weighted imaging and high signal on T2-weighted imaging. Mineralization of the lobules can be identified on MR imaging, particularly on gradient-echo sequences. The areas of calcification produce a distinctive speckled pattern of low signal within the lesion on T2-weighted images. On the high-resolution images, the low signal within the areas of calcification can appear clustered at the periphery of the cartilage lobules. Mature enchondromata that have undergone endochondral ossification often demonstrate small areas of marrow fat located centrally in the cartilage lobules (1). Presence of this heterotopic fat produces a pattern of speckled high signal on the T1-weighted images. In one large series of enchondroma, this finding was present in 65% of cases. Contrast enhancement is classically present in a "rings and arcs" pattern, as seen in this example (3).

REFERENCES

1. Murphey MD, Flemming DJ, Boyea SR, et al. Enchondroma versus chondrosarcoma in the appendicular skeleton: differentiating features. *Radiographics* 1998;18:1213–1237.
2. Takigawa K. Chondroma of the bones of the hand. *J Bone Joint Surg [Am]* 1971;53:1591–1599.
3. Aoki J, Sone S, Fujioka F, et al. MR of enchondroma and chondrosarcoma: rings and arcs of Gd-DTPA enhancement. *JCAT* 1991;15:1011–1016.
4. Schwartz HS, Zimmerman NB, Simon MA, et al. The malignant potential of enchondromatosis. *J Bone Joint Surg [Am]* 1987;69:269–274.

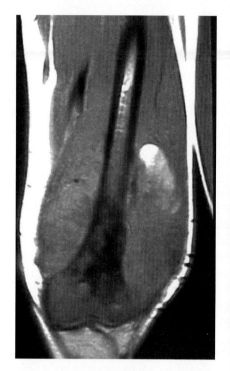

FIGURE 9.95A

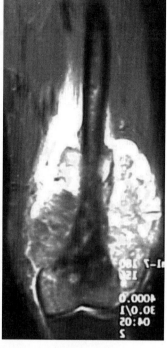

FIGURE 9.95B

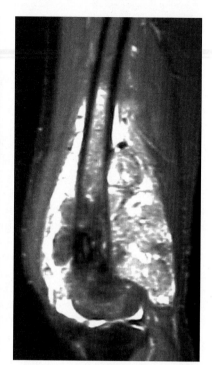

FIGURE 9.95C

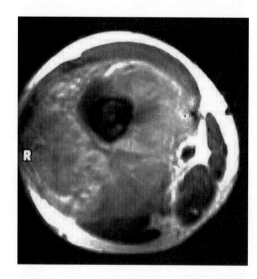

FIGURE 9.95D

CLINICAL HISTORY

A 25-year-old male developed a rapidly growing painful mass in his right leg.

FINDINGS

T1-weighted and STIR coronal images show a long area of abnormal bone marrow infiltration in the distal right femur, with extension of the intraosseous lesion into the adjacent soft tissues (Fig. 9.95A–B). The tumor is low signal on the T1-weighted sequence and becomes more heterogeneous on the STIR sequence, though the intraosseous component exhibits lower signal than the soft-tissue component. The superolateral portion of the soft tissue is high signal on the T1-weighted and STIR images, consistent with intratumoral hemorrhage. The sagittal STIR image (Fig. 9.95C) shows the longitudinal extent of the lesion, as well as a small effusion within the adjacent knee joint. An axial proton-density-weighted image shows low signal within the bone, cortical irregularity, and a large heterogeneous mass surrounding the distal femur (Fig. 9.95D).

DIAGNOSIS

Osteogenic sarcoma (osteosarcoma) of the distal femur.

DISCUSSION

Osteosarcoma is the most common primary malignant tumor of bone in patients under the age of 30, representing approximately 15% of all primary bone malignancies (1). Males are affected twice as frequently as females (2). Osteosarcoma is classified by its histologic subtype, by its grade, or by the location of the lesion in the longitudinal and transverse axes of the bone. The high-grade intramedullary variant of osteogenic sarcoma, which typically arises in the metaphysis of the long bones of the lower extremity, is the most common form (1). Since osteosarcoma is highly aggressive and rapidly growing, with doubling times of 20 to 30 days, the tumor is typically larger than 5 cm at the time of diagnosis (1). Characteristic radiographic findings are an aggressive metaphyseal lesion with a wide zone of transition, showing mixed lysis and sclerosis within the bone, immature periostitis, and formation of cloudlike mineralized osteoid in the soft tissues (2).

The prognosis for osteosarcoma has improved in the past two decades with the development of limb-sparing surgical procedures and adjuvant therapies, resulting in improved functional outcome and 5-year survival rates of 55% to 70% (3). The presence of metastasis, local extent of the tumor, invasion of the adjacent articulation or neurovascular structures, and response of the tumor to preoperative chemotherapy or radiation are all important factors in determining the most appropriate surgical procedure and for establishing the prognosis of the lesion. Cross-sectional imaging is employed routinely for preoperative staging and for monitoring tumor response (3,4).

Although the diagnosis of osteosarcoma can usually be established with conventional radiographs, MR imaging plays an important role in staging the anatomic extent of the tumor. On MR imaging, osteosarcoma typically shows signal heterogeneity due to the mixture of bone sclerosis, active tumor tissue, necrosis, and hemorrhage. Areas of extensive bone sclerosis or tumor mineralization appear as low signal on all imaging sequences. Areas of intralesional hemorrhages, which appear as regions of high signal on the T1- and T2-weighted images, are common in both the osseous and the soft-tissue portions of the lesion (1). Peritumoral edema can be pronounced in the bone and soft tissues, leading to overstaging of the extent of the lesion (3). Contrast enhancement, quantitative assessment of perfusion, and diffusion-weighted imaging may help in increasing the accuracy of staging, particularly following preoperative adjuvant therapy (3,4).

REFERENCES

1. Murphey MD, Robbin MR, McRae GA, et al. The many faces of osteosarcoma. *Radiographics* 1997;17:1205–1231.
2. Logan PM, Mitchell MJ, Munk PL. Imaging of variant osteosarcoma with an emphasis on CT and MR imaging. *AJR* 1998;171:1531–1537.
3. Schima W, Amman G, Stiglbauer R, et al. Preoperative staging of osteosarcoma: efficacy of MR imaging in detecting joint involvement. *AJR* 1994;163:1171–1175.
4. Lang P, Wendland MF, Saeed M, et al. Osteogenic sarcoma: noninvasive *in vivo* assessment of tumor necrosis with diffusion-weighted MR imaging. *Radiology* 1998;206:227–235.

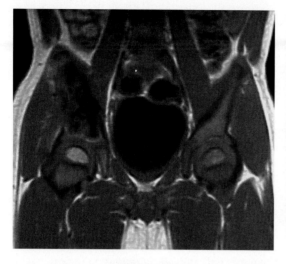

FIGURE 9.96A   **FIGURE 9.96B**

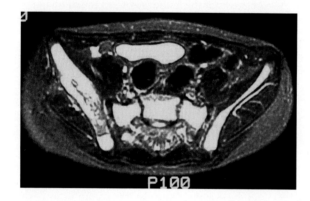

FIGURE 9.96C

CLINICAL HISTORY

This 2-year-old boy developed a limp and refused to bear weight on his right leg.

FINDINGS

The coronal T1-weighted MR of the pelvis (Fig. 9.96A) shows abnormal bone marrow in the right ileum above the acetabulum. The iliac bone marrow is inhomogeneous and lower signal than normal, and the bony cortex appears irregular. The corresponding inversion recovery image (Fig. 9.96B) shows high signal within the abnormal ileum, as well as abnormal signal in the soft tissues adjacent to the diseased bone. The fat-suppressed axial T2-weighted image (Fig. 9.96C) highlights the asymmetry in the iliac bone and shows patchy cortical destruction of the bone with an adjacent soft-tissue mass.

DIAGNOSIS

Ewing sarcoma of the right iliac bone.

DISCUSSION

After osteosarcoma, Ewing sarcoma is the most common skeletal malignancy of childhood, representing an estimated 10% of all primary malignancies of bone (1). Undifferentiated Ewing sarcoma, which can arise in either bone or the soft tissues, is related to a better-differentiated tumor known as the primitive neuroectodermal tumor (or PNET), and these two lesions are now considered as parts of the spectrum of a single pathologic entity (2). The osseous form of Ewing sarcoma is characteristically found in the diaphyseal or metadiaphyseal region of the long bones, though involvement of the flat bones of the pelvis and chest wall is not uncommon (1). Of all cases of Ewing sarcoma entered in the Intergroup Ewing's Sarcoma Study (IESS), 21% of these malignancies arose in the flat bones of the pelvis (3).

The radiographic features of Ewing sarcoma are those of a poorly marginated, permeative lytic lesion of bone showing aggressive periosteal new bone formation, such as the spiculated or hair-on-end patterns of periostitis, surrounded by a disproportionately large soft-tissue mass. Intramedullary and cortical sclerosis of the bone can be seen in up to a third of cases (3). The soft-tissue component of Ewing sarcoma is due to the tumor's ability to spread rapidly through the Haversian canals of the bony cortex without causing macroscopic cortical destruction (3). The presence of a large soft-tissue mass adjacent to a relatively normal-appearing cortex is one of the hallmarks of osseous Ewing sarcoma.

On MR imaging, the infiltrated bone marrow shows low signal on T1-weighted images and increases in signal on T2 weighting. Invasion of the cortex, which is a common feature of Ewing tumor, is well seen on MR as the low-signal cortex is replaced by the infiltrating higher-signal neoplasm (4). The soft-tissue component that typically accompanies Ewing sarcoma is well seen on MR, with better visualization than can be obtained with CT (4). The signal within the soft-tissue component of Ewing sarcoma is variable, though it is often higher than the intraosseous component on the T2-weighted images.

REFERENCES

1. Buck JL. Primary Ewing sarcoma of rib. *Radiographics* 1990;10:899–914.
2. Mueller DL, Grant RM, Riding MD, et al. Cortical saucerization: an unusual imaging finding of Ewing sarcoma. *AJR* 1994;163:401–403.
3. Reinus WR, Gilula LA. Radiology of Ewing's sarcoma: Intergroup Ewing's Sarcoma Study (IESS). *Radiographics* 1984;4:929–944.
4. Boyko OB, Cory DA, Cohen MD, et al. MR imaging of osteogenic and Ewing's sarcoma. *AJR* 1987;148:317–322.

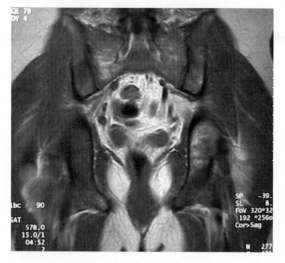

FIGURE 9.97A

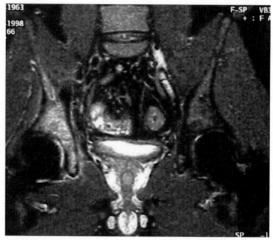

FIGURE 9.97B

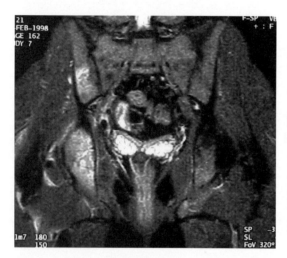

FIGURE 9.97C

FIGURE 9.97D

CLINICAL HISTORY

This 36-year-old man complained of fatigue, shortness of breath, and easy bruising. His initial hematologic work-up showed numerous abnormalities, and he was referred for MR imaging to select a suitable location for bone marrow biopsy.

FINDINGS

Coronal T1-weighted images (Fig. 9.97A–B) of the pelvis obtained at the level of the posterior acetabulum (A) and the acetabular roof (B) show multiple large areas of low-signal tissue replacing the normal fatty bone marrow. A large lesion is present in the right supraacetabular region, with smaller le-sions located in the right ileum adjacent to the sacroiliac joint and in the left inferior pubic ramus. The corresponding STIR images (Fig. 9.97C–D) show high signal in the corre-sponding regions of abnormal marrow. The cortex of the bone appears normal and there is no soft-tissue component.

DIAGNOSIS

Acute myelogenous leukemia.

DISCUSSION

Leukemia is a primary hematologic malignancy arising directly from the reticulum cells of the bone marrow rather than from its supporting mesenchymal elements (1). Leukemia can arise at any age and is a common malignancy in both the young and the elderly. Many forms of leukemia are recognized, based on the clinical presentation and the histologic characteristics of the malignant cells. Acute leukemia occurs in both adults and children, but the chronic form of leukemia is much more common in adults. In children, the most common histologic forms of leukemia are either the acute lymphocytic or the acute undifferentiated forms (1). Chronic granulocytic leukemia typically is seen in the middle-aged adult, whereas chronic lymphocytic leukemia is most common in the elderly patient. Whereas the acute leukemias often have a fulminant course, the clinical course in the chronic leukemias is often indolent (2). Treatment of the leukemias has improved dramatically in the last two decades with the advent of ablative chemotherapy and bone marrow transplantation.

Three patterns of marrow infiltration have been described in patients with leukemia: diffuse uniform, diffuse patchy, and focal (3). Diffuse infiltrative leukemia is typically associated with the chronic forms of leukemia. Although the patchy and focal forms are easily identified on MR images, the diffuse uniform pattern may be difficult to recognize, especially with spin-echo sequences. The appearance of the diffuse uniform pattern has been termed the *flip-flop sign* (4). On MR images, there is a diffuse decrease in the marrow signal intensity on T1-weighted spin-echo images, with an increase in signal intensity on T2-weighted spin-echo images, a pattern opposite that of normal fatty marrow. The MR changes can be absent or very subtle in early diffuse leukemia, and marrow abnormalities may not be visible during the early stages of the disease. Even using advanced techniques such as quantitative MR imaging, significant T1 shortening of the bone marrow can be detected in less than half of patients with early-stage chronic lymphocytic leukemia (2).

The diffuse patchy and focal forms of leukemic infiltration of the bone marrow are more easily recognized. Multifocal lesions are typically present, usually limited to the bone marrow space without cortical disruption. Leukemia results in loss of the normal high-signal fatty marrow on the T1-weighted images. The disease has a highly variable appearance on T2 sequences and often does not show as much increased signal as would be expected from the alterations seen on the T1-weighted images. Leukemic infiltrates are typically isointense or mildly hyperintense compared with the normal bone marrow on the T2-weighted sequence (5). In approximately 5% of patients with acute leukemia, aggressive focal lesions that produce localized regions of osteolytic bone destruction are identified. These focal masslike lesions of leukemic cells are known as granulocytic sarcoma but are sometimes still referred to by their historic name, *chloroma*, named for their greenish coloration on macroscopic examination (6). The granulocytic sarcoma, like diffuse and patchy leukemic infiltration, may not show much hyperintensity on T2 weighting, though the lesions do tend to enhance avidly following intravenous gadolinium enhancement (6).

REFERENCES

1. Pear BL. Skeletal manifestations of the lymphomas and leukemias. *Semin Roentgenol* 1974;9:229–240.
2. Lecouvet FE, Vande Berg BC, Michaux L, et al. Early chronic lymphocytic leukemia: prognostic value of quantitative bone marrow MR imaging findings and correlation with hematologic variables. *Radiology* 1997;204:813–818.
3. Bohndorf K, Benz-Bohm G, Gross-Fengels W, et al. MRI of the knee region in leukemic children: Part I. Initial pattern in patients with untreated disease. *Pediatr Radiol* 1990;20:179–183.
4. Ruzal-Shapiro C, Berdon WE, Cohen MD, et al. MR imaging of diffuse bone marrow replacement in pediatric patients with cancer. *Radiology* 1991;181:587–589.
5. McKinstry CS, Steiner RE, Young AT, et al. Bone marrow in leukemia and aplastic anemia: MR imaging before, during, and after treatment. *Radiology* 1987;162:701–707.
6. Pui MH, Fletcher BD, Langston JW. Granulocytic sarcoma in childhood leukemia: imaging features. *Radiology* 1994;190:698–702.

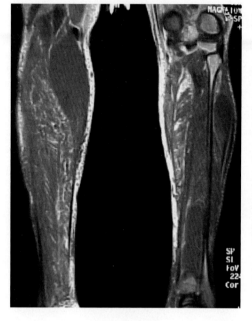

FIGURE 9.98A

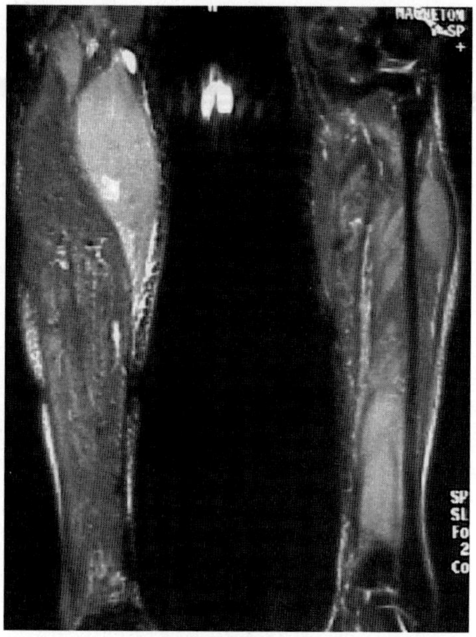

FIGURE 9.98B

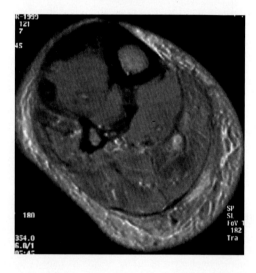

FIGURE 9.98C

CLINICAL HISTORY

This 82-year-old man was referred by his oncologist because he was developing pain and swelling of both lower legs.

FINDINGS

A coronal T1-weighted image (Fig. 9.98A) of both legs shows loss of the normal fatty septations within the muscles of both lower legs. The STIR image (Fig. 9.98B) shows abnormal increased signal within the medial head of the gastrocnemius muscle in the right leg and within the soleus and peroneal muscles on the left. An axial T2-weighted image (Fig. 9.98C) of the right midcalf shows mild hyperintensity within multiple muscles, with abnormal muscle in the anterior, lateral, and posterior compartments of the calf. Despite these widespread signal abnormalities, there does not appear to be significant mass effect. There is stranding and edema within the subcutaneous tissues. The bone appears normal.

DIAGNOSIS

Non-Hodgkin's lymphoma of skeletal muscle.

DISCUSSION

While the etiology of lymphoma remains uncertain, it is well recognized that patients with immune system deficiency due to conditions such as congenital immunodeficiency, AIDS, or chemotherapy-induced immunosuppression have a significantly increased risk for developing lymphoma compared with the general population (1). Lymphoma is subclassified into Hodgkin's disease and the non-Hodgkin's lymphomas. The non-Hodgkin's lymphomas, which are four times more common than Hodgkin's disease, are a heterogeneous group of disorders that account for 3% of all newly diagnosed cancers in the United States (1).

Primary lymphoma can involve any portion of the musculoskeletal system, including bone (reticulum cell sarcoma), skin and subcutaneous tissues (mycosis fungoides), and muscle (2). Primary lymphoma of the musculoskeletal system is much less common than secondary involvement by primary nodal or visceral lymphoma. Secondary musculoskeletal involvement can develop either via hematogenous spread or by contiguous extension of lymphoma from adjacent lymph nodes or viscera.

Lymphomatous involvement of muscle is uncommon, presenting in less than 2% of patients with lymphoma (3). Muscular lymphoma can be the primary site of disease, but more commonly, muscle lymphoma represents a metastatic focus in a patient with widely disseminated disease (2). Both primary and secondary lymphomas of the muscle are typically due to non-Hodgkin's lymphoma. Neoplastic involvement can present as a discrete mass or as a diffuse tumor infiltration; the latter pattern is more common (2). The most common sites of muscular lymphoma are the large muscles of the lower extremity, particularly the anterior muscles of the thigh and the posterior muscles of the calf (3). Differentiation of primary from secondary muscle involvement is difficult based on the local appearance of the lesion. The diagnosis of primary muscular lymphoma requires exclusion of systemic or nodal disease in the remainder of the body (3).

On MR imaging, lymphoma of the muscle is typically quite extensive at presentation, as it infiltrates diffusely throughout the muscle. The tumor typically infiltrates a long segment of the extremity and frequently involves multiple muscles. Multiple muscle involvement is common because lymphoma spreads by infiltration of individual malignant cells, resulting in a pattern of growth that readily violates fascia boundaries (4). Mass effect is not a prominent feature.

The areas of lymphomatous involvement are isointense or hypointense to the normal muscle on the T1-weighted sequences. The tumor increases in signal on the T2-weighted sequences, showing signal similar to slightly greater than the subcutaneous fat. Marked signal hyperintensity on the T2-weighted images, as is typically present in most mesenchymal soft-tissue neoplasms, is not a feature of muscular lymphoma. Diffuse enhancement is seen following intravenous gadolinium administration (3). Subcutaneous stranding or soft-tissue nodules extending into the subcutaneous tissues may be present, as well as adjacent bony involvement (3,4). Although these MR features are not specific, the diagnosis should be considered when a large infiltrative lesion, without prominent mass effect or marked T2 hyperintensity, is identified in the deep muscles of the lower extremity. Definitive diagnosis can be established by needle biopsy of the lesion.

Submitted by Lai-No Chiu-Serodio, The Good Samaritan Hospital, Lebanon, PA.

REFERENCES

1. Castellino RA. The non-Hodkin lymphomas: practical concepts for the diagnostic radiologist. *Radiology* 1991;178:315–321.
2. Malloy PC, Fishman EK, Magid D. Lymphoma of bone, muscle, and skin: CT findings. *AJR* 1992;159:805–809.
3. Lee VS, Martinez S, Coleman RE. Primary muscle lymphoma: clinical and imaging findings. *Radiology* 1997;203:237–244.
4. Chew RS, Schellingerhout D, Keel SB. Primary lymphoma of skeletal muscle. *AJR* 1999;172:1370.

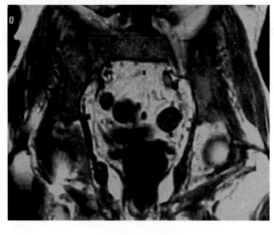

FIGURE 9.99A

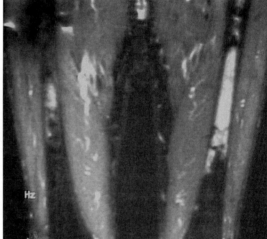

FIGURE 9.99B

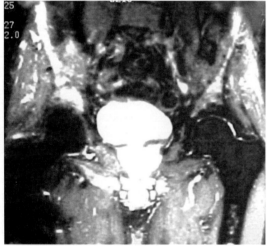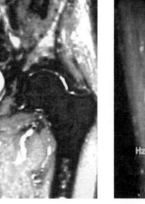

FIGURE 9.99C

FIGURE 9.99D

CLINICAL HISTORY

A 72-year-old male complained of generalized bone pain. His serum electrophoresis showed a monoclonal gammopathy.

FINDINGS

T1-weighted coronal images of the pelvis (Fig. 9.99A) and femora (Fig. 9.99B) show multiple large focal areas of marrow replacement by low-signal intramedullary lesions. Metallic artifact at the right hip joint is from a prior hip replacement. The STIR coronal image (Fig. 9.99C) of the pelvis at the level of the hip joints show multiple foci of high signal within the bone marrow. Widespread replacement of the bone marrow is present. The coronal STIR image of the proximal femora (Fig. 9.99D) also shows multiple well-demarcated osseous lesions.

DIAGNOSIS

Multiple myeloma.

DISCUSSION

Multiple myeloma is a primary bone marrow malignancy caused by focal, disseminated, or diffuse infiltration of the marrow by a monoclonal proliferation of malignant plasma cells of reticuloendothelial origin (1). The peak incidence of multiple myeloma is in the elderly patient, typically presenting in the sixth or seventh decade (1). Initial complaints are nonspecific and include fatigue, weakness, and nonspecific bone pain (2). Later in the course of the disease, pathologic fractures can develop due to widespread bone demineralization. Vertebral compression fractures develop in 55% to 70% of patients with myeloma and are most common in the thoracic and thoracolumbar regions (3). The most specific laboratory finding in multiple myeloma is the presence of an abnormal serum and/or urine electrophoresis (4). Blind biopsy of the bone marrow or directed biopsy of focal lesions is typically obtained for confirmation of the diagnosis.

Two main patterns of marrow involvement can be recognized on histologic evaluation: a diffuse homogeneous infiltrative pattern and a more focal pattern of larger nodules (4). The infiltrative pattern of multiple myeloma does not destroy trabecular or cortical bone in its initial stages, making it difficult to detect on conventional radiography (1). Radiographs can be normal or demonstrate osseous demineralization. Scintigraphy is insensitive because the tumor cells incite minimal adjacent bone response. CT shows osteopenia and increased attenuation of the bone marrow, but the findings are very subtle and easily overlooked unless focal destructive lesions have complicated the disease. MR is more sensitive but a significant number of patients with early multiple myeloma are still overlooked. Even though MR imaging generally shows very high sensitivity for marrow disorders, marrow infiltration by myeloma is difficult to recognize in the infiltrative form of the disease.

With standard spin-echo imaging, 6% to 34% of multiple myeloma patients have a normal MR examination, even in the presence of widespread marrow disease and pathologic vertebral fractures (1,4–6). Fractured vertebra can appear benign on MR imaging in up to 59% of patients with myeloma-induced compression deformities of the vertebral body (3). T1-weighted images are only moderately sensitive, showing focal lesions in 25% to 31% and a variegated, inhomogeneous, or diffuse decrease in bone marrow signal in 38% to 53% of cases (1,5,6). On T2-weighted images, focal nodules of high signal intensity can be seen in more than 50% of patients with multiple myeloma (1,5). In the remaining patients, the T2-weighted images show persistent low- or intermediate-signal marrow that is difficult to recognize as abnormal. The nodules of myeloma are more conspicuous on STIR images, where they demonstrate uniform high signal (6). Multiple myeloma enhances homogeneously following intravenous gadolinium administration, but contrast enhancement does not increase the sensitivity of MR for detection of infiltrative myeloma (6). The focal nodular form of myeloma is more readily recognized. In this form, multiple larger nodules of myeloma are seen superimposed on a background of normal marrow. Patients with the focal nodular form tend to have lower marrow plasmacytosis and cellularity than patients with the infiltrative pattern (4). These nodules of malignant cells are dark on the T1-weighted images and increase in signal on T2-weighted or STIR images. The focal nodular form is often difficult to distinguish from metastatic disease solely on the basis of imaging examination.

REFERENCES

1. Libshitz HI, Malthouse SR, Cunningham D, et al. Multiple myeloma. Appearance at MR imaging. *Radiology* 1992;182:833–837.
2. Rahmouni A, Divine M, Mathieu D, et al. MR appearance of multiple myeloma of the spine before and after treatment. *AJR* 1993;160:1053–1057.
3. Lecouvet FE, Vande Berg BC, Maldague BE, et al. Vertebral compression fractures in multiple myeloma: Part 1. Distribution and appearance at MR imaging. *Radiology* 1997;204:195–199.
4. Lecouvet FE, Vande Berg BC, Michaux L, et al. Stage III multiple myeloma: clinical and prognostic value of spinal bone marrow imaging. *Radiology* 1998;209:653–660.
5. Moulopoulos LA, Varma DGK, Dimopoulos MA, et al. Multiple myeloma: spinal MR imaging in patients with untreated newly diagnosed disease. *Radiology* 1992;185:833–840.
6. Rahmouni A, Divine M, Mathieu D, et al. Detection of multiple myeloma involving the spine: efficacy of fat-suppression and contrast-enhanced MR imaging. *AJR* 1993;160:1049–1052.

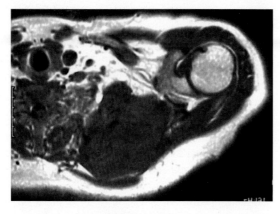

FIGURE 9.100A

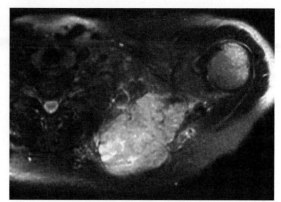

FIGURE 9.100B

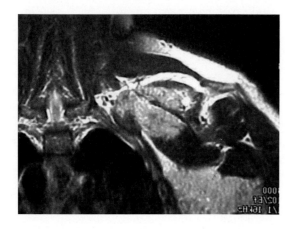

FIGURE 9.100C-1

CLINICAL HISTORY

A 56-year-old man with a history of renal cell carcinoma developed severe pain in his right scapular region. A radionuclide bone scan showed a solitary focus of increased accumulation in the right scapula.

FINDINGS

The axial T1-weighted image (Fig. 9.100A) of the right shoulder obtained at the level of the coracoid process shows a low-signal mass replacing the body of the scapula with extension into the soft tissues. On the corresponding axial fat-suppressed T2-weighted image (Fig. 9.100B), the high-signal soft-tissue component is easier to differentiate from the adjacent low-signal muscle. The coronal T2-weighted image shows the large soft-tissue component surrounding the spine of the scapula (Fig. 9.100C-2, *arrow*) and elevating the trapezius muscle (Fig. 9.100C-2, *arrowhead*).

DIAGNOSIS

Metastatic disease from renal cell carcinoma involving the scapula.

DISCUSSION

Metastatic disease to bone is far more common than primary malignancy of the skeleton. In fact, metastasis is the most common neoplastic disease of bone in all age groups, but particularly in the elderly patient, in whom metastasis to bone far outnumbers primary bone malignancy (1). The most common primary malignancies to metastasize to the skeleton include carcinoma of the lung, breast, prostate, kidney, and thyroid (2). Together, these primary malignancies account for more than 75% of all metastases in adults. Metastases from renal cell carcinoma tend to be highly vascular and rapidly growing, and are often associated with a prominent soft-tissue mass.

Because of its ability to image the whole skeleton rapidly and inexpensively, scintigraphy is typically utilized as the initial screening examination for the detection of metastatic disease in a patient with a known primary malignancy. MR is more sensitive than scintigraphy for the detection of metastatic disease to bone, but MR cannot be used to evaluate the entire skeleton at one setting (3). Frank et al. reviewed a large series of patients with metastatic disease and found that MR and scintigraphy had equivalent accuracy in most patients, but MR detected significantly more lesions than the bone scan in a significant minority (4). The advantage of MR is particularly evident for infiltrative neoplasms such as multiple myeloma and lymphoma, which may have normal scintigrams in the presence of widespread disease. MR is frequently obtained to determine the nature of a scintigraphic abnormality, particularly if it is solitary or indeterminate on the bone scan. MR imaging is also commonly employed to determine the size and extent of a known metastatic lesion and to determine its relationship to adjacent neurovascular structures before surgical debridement or radiation therapy.

Metastases to the skeleton can be solitary, can be disseminated, or can diffusely involve the bone marrow (5). Metastatic disease to bone presents as a solitary lesion in 10% to 15% of patients (2). The most common pattern of skeletal metastasis is the disseminated pattern, with multiple areas of tumor separated by regions of normal bone marrow. The diffuse pattern shows metastatic disease throughout the skeleton. The solitary and disseminated patterns are easily detected on MR imaging. The diffuse pattern is more problematic, and differentiation of subtle diffuse infiltration from prominent hematopoietic marrow may be difficult.

On MR imaging, metastases appear as low signal within the bone marrow on T1-weighted images. The signal within a metastasis is typically less than that of the intervertebral disk and muscle, whereas normal marrow is higher signal than these normal structures. The signal of metastatic disease on T2-weighted images is more variable and depends upon the nature of the adjacent bony response. Lytic tumors show high signal, whereas sclerotic lesions may appear hypointense, hyperintense, or isointense to normal bone marrow, depending on the extent of bone sclerosis.

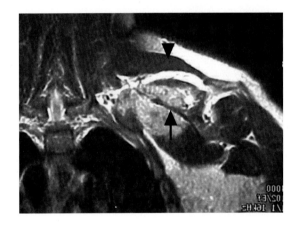

FIGURE 9.100C-2

REFERENCES

1. Resnick D, Niwayama G. Skeletal metastasis. In: Resnick D, Niwayama G, eds. *Diagnosis of bone and joint disorders,* 3rd ed. Philadelphia: WB Saunders, 1995:3991–4064.
2. Thrall JH, Ellis BI. Skeletal metastases. *Radiol Clin North Am* 1987;25:1155.
3. Algra PR, Bloem JL, Tissing H, et al. Detection of vertebral metastases: comparison between MR imaging and bone scintigraphy. *Radiographics* 1991;11:219–232.
4. Frank JA, Ling A, Patronas NJ, et al. Detection of malignant bone tumors: MR imaging vs scintigraphy. *AJR* 1990;155:1043–1048.
5. Pathria MN, Isaacs P. Magnetic resonance imaging of bone marrow. *Curr Opin Radiol* 1992;4:21–31.

INDEX

Page numbers followed by an f refer to figures.